Sixty Years In Search Of Cures
An Herbalist's Success With Chinese Herbs

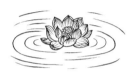

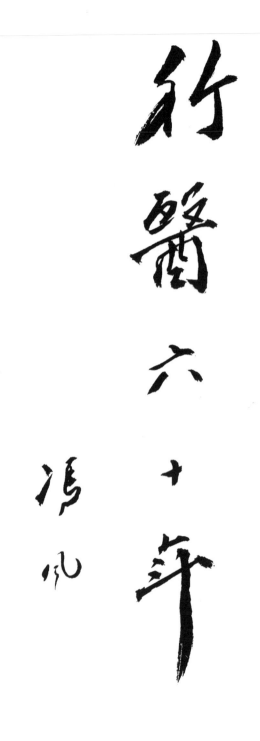

行醫六十年

馮凡

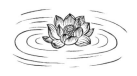

Sixty Years In Search Of Cures
An Herbalist's Success With Chinese Herbs

by

Dr. Fung Fung
& John Fung

Get Well Foundation
Dublin, California

North Atlantic Books
Berkeley, California

Disclaimer

The following information is intended for general information purposes only. Individuals with a health problem should always see their health care provider before administering any suggestions made in this book. Any application of the material set forth in the following pages is at the reader's discretion and sole responsibility.

Sixty Years in Search of Cures

Published by:
Get Well Foundation
7172 Regional St. #116
Dublin, CA 94568-2324

Distributed by:
North Atlantic Books
P.O. Box 12327
Berkeley, CA 94701

Cover art and design by Bruce Wang
Book design and production by Catherine E. Campaigne
Copy editing by Nissi Wang and Andrew Gaeddert

Sixty Years in Search of Cures is published by Get Well Foundation, a non-profit organization whose purpose is to educate the public and health care providers about natural therapies that are complements to Western medicine. Publications, classes, symposia, and community-based research projects are planned.

ISBN 0–9638285–1–7 : $15.95

How to Order:

Single copies may be ordered from Get Well Foundation, 7172 Regional St, #116, Dublin, CA 94568-2324.

For trade, bookstore, and wholesale inquiries, contact North Atlantic Books, P.O. Box 12327, Berkeley, CA 94701.

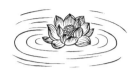

This book is dedicated to those who suffer from physical ailments and emotional distress.

Acknowledgments

Our gratitude goes to all the patients who have come to us for medical help. Their trust and faith in us and in Chinese herbs have made healing them much easier. Their cooperation has provided valuable information for broadening our knowledge and deepening our expertise. Many patients have become our friends, and their encouragement has given us enough reason to write this book.

We would like to thank Andrew Gaeddert, an herbalist and author. His comments enabled us to make many refinements to the manuscript.

The writing of this book would have been much more difficult if it were not for the constant support of our family, especially Christina, who assisted in the verification of the medical information contained in this book. We are greatly indebted to her.

Contents

Foreword
Robert Johns, O. M.D., L.Ac.

Dr. Fung has been my friend and mentor for over fourteen years. Although I cannot remember any particular time that I became his student, I can clearly remember the day when I realized that I had been his student for some time. This beginning set the tone for my future studies with Dr. Fung. There are many facets of diagnosis and prescription that weren't obvious as I was learning them. Over time I have come to understand that one of the most valuable tools I gained from my studies with Dr. Fung was an ability to see the world through his eyes. By understanding his world view, I learned that Chinese medicine is not just the application of a collection of facts called knowledge, but the whole configuration of the thinking that goes into Chinese medicine. To see in this way is to be able to take skills of diagnosing and prescribing to a more profound level.

I remember the time when a woman brought her infant to see Dr. Fung. The child's condition was serious, one that required longterm treatment. After they left, Dr. Fung asked me, "Did you notice anything unusual about the mother?" Without waiting for an answer, Dr. Fung continued, "I prescribed only the best herbs," he said. "The mother was closer than usual to her child and if I hadn't prescribed the best herbs I would have lost her confidence. She wouldn't come back and I wouldn't be able to continue treating her baby." For the Chinese, health and the practice of medicine are part of the interweaving of the fabric of our lives, not something separate. To be involved in the practice of Chinese medine is to be involved in life. The greater one's involvement and understanding of life, the greater is one's ability to diagnose and treat. Looking back at all my time in Dr. Fung's clinic, there never was a day that he did not have a new way of saying what he had to teach. Sometimes, what he had to say did not seem directly related to Chinese medicine. In retrospect, I saw that Dr. Fung found ways to affect my thinking and orientation to the world around me, and thereby affected my thinking and orientation as a physician.

To say that Dr. Fung's understanding of prescribing is extensive is a great understatement. His office was in the back of an herb store owned by a Mr. Liu, who was trained as an herbalist by his father and grandfather and whose own knowledge of Chinese herbs is considerable. Once, I was watching Mr. Liu fill a prescription by Dr. Fung which contained a number of unusual herbs, and I asked if he had had to stock additional herbs after Dr. Fung set up office in his store. "Yes," was his reply, "about four or five hundred herbs."

A side of Dr. Fung that he did not let his patients see is that he studies every day. Each day he studies one herb, all its possible uses, and its combination with other herbs. His love of Chinese herbs and his unrelenting commitment to improving his skills is part of what makes him so great.

Foreword
Robert N. Dreyfuss, O.M.D., L.Ac.

I was Dr. Fung's "indoor" student from 1984 until his retirement at the end of 1992. The training I received was traditional: I sat at his desk in the herb store while he saw patients, often forty to sixty in a given day on a first come first served basis. He would ask questions, feel the pulses, look at the tongue, and then write the prescription in a beautiful flowing hand, which he would share with me in Cantonese. When there was time, I could ask questions or he would comment on an interesting aspect of the patient's case.

Dr. Fung is fluent in several languages, and had many patients who came to him because of his lingual versatility as well as his considerable reputation in the community. Because I unfortunately do not share his command of Cantonese, Mandarin, and Vietnamese, I often did not have a clear understanding of the patients' complaints nor of Dr. Fung's comments and advice to them.

For any given case, Dr. Fung might or might not explain his prescribing rationale. He wanted me to work for the knowledge and underlying principles of his formulas. When Dr. Fung realized I was truly committed to learning the intricacies of Chinese herbal medicine with him, little pearls would be shared as to an herb's subtle uses and its functions in a formula. Much of the information I received was not available in texts, and his extraordinary command of the pharmacopia greatly expanded what I had been taught in Chinese medical college, and revealed the paucity of the herbal curriculum considered sufficient for practicing. All Dr. Fung wanted was that I show interest, ask questions, and study. Through the years I have utilized what he taught me, and was able to bring cases to him for consultation. From visits to his home, I saw that even after sixty years of practice, Dr. Fung kept a book on herbs next to his bed and another in his bathroom, and that he studied daily. I shall always be grateful to him for his generosity and knowledge, both personally and in my medical practice.

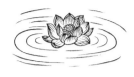

Introduction

The Quest For Alternative Medicine

It was another great milestone for Western medicine when Christiaan Barnard successfully performed the first human heart transplant in December 1967. Western medicine had once again electrified the world with its progress and specialization. It seemed destined to become the universal medicine accepted by all cultures.

Today, the technological advances of Western medicine continue to dazzle the world, but America is facing enormous health care problems brought to public attention by the Clinton administration. As a reform bill is being drafted and debated, the costs of health care continue to soar. At the same time, the quality of health care does not appear to show any significant improvement.

Western medicine has reached an important crossroad in America. It is very advanced, but it is also very expensive. It should benefit every citizen, but so many cannot even afford to pay the insurance premiums. It should have developed permanent cures for various illnesses, but so many people find themselves increasingly dependent on drugs to stay healthy. The rapidly rising costs of health care are drowning both public and private employers. Many corporations are now requiring their employees to shoulder a greater share of the health care expense.

With this reality in mind, my father and I decided to write a book on alternative medicine. We want to promote a better understanding of Chinese herbal medicine as a low-cost alternative with minimum side effects. Chinese medicine emphasizes prevention and natural cure by restoring or maintaining the balance of body functions. In contrast, Western medicine with its modern technology, stresses human intervention to cure an illness. While Western medicine has captured the limelight in all areas including technology and cost, Chinese medicine is content with perfecting the art of living in balance and harmony with nature, something that is subtle but essential for healthy life.

Because of the gulf that exists in theory and technology, Western and Chinese medicines are likely to go their separate ways, thus widening the divergence between them even further. Nevertheless, both disciplines have one commonality: to alleviate human suffering. Given this common purpose, the two have many complementarities. This book highlights the areas where Chinese medicine can complement Western medicine in order to reduce costs and produce a natural cure that has few side effects.

My father has been a practitioner of Chinese medicine for sixty years in four different places: Canton (now Guangzhou), Saigon (now Ho Chi Minh City), Hong Kong, and San Francisco. Since our family immigrated to America in 1979, other immigrants from Vietnam and Hong Kong have found him again in San Francisco. Apart from this large Asian clientele, he has gained credibility with an increasing number of native-born Americans who have discovered the benefits and cost-effectiveness of Chinese medicine. In addition, for many years, my father has been offering free lessons and guidance to a group of acupuncturists and herbalists in the San Francisco Bay Area.

Many patients and students are enthusiastic to learn more about Chinese medicine. Presently, there are many English-language works about Chinese herbs and medical theory. We want to make a contribution in other areas, such as prevention, diagnosis, therapy, and practice. Apart from satisfying the enthusiasm of patients and students, we hope to arouse the interest of the American public who have never experienced the benefits of Chinese medicine.

Writing about Chinese medicine for a Western culture faces the twin hurdles of credibility and acceptability. It is only natural that many Westerners harbor doubts or disbeliefs about Chinese medicine. Part of the reason is that it is simply foreign or little known. Therefore, in this book we concentrate on the real-life stories about people and their illnesses, and the herbs and methods employed to heal them. While readers may not understand a foreign culture, they should have no problem in empathizing with those who have suffered and have been healed. (To preserve confidentiality, fictitious names of patients are used in the case histories.)

In the summer of 1968, I left Hong Kong for college in America. When young, I had never been treated by a Western doctor before except for inoculations and physical examinations required by my schools. I had grown up under the protection of Chinese herbs (and of course my parents), a fact that I had long taken for granted.

My first winter in America was very special. It was the first time I ever saw snow. One afternoon, some friends and I played in the freshly fallen snow outside our dormitory at Washington State University. We were not wearing any heavy clothing. The next morning I could not get out of bed. My joints ached, I felt extremely fatigued, and was short of breath. My friends had to carry me to the hospital. After two days of testing and appointments with various specialists, I was told that my case was an enigma, but that it could be rheumatoid arthritis. I was hospitalized for a week while the doctors administered treatment and observed the results.

On the day that I was released, I was apprehensive about the bill and asked the nurse at the registration desk how much money I owed. "Don't worry! Your insurance company will take care of everything." This was the first time I had benefited from insurance. I had always seen patients paying my father in cash after each treatment. Now, I could see that health insurance was a great benefactor since I did not have to pay a cent for my hospital stay.

I was told by my doctors that the arthritis could flare up again, and that if it did, I should take the prescribed capsules, which contained cortisone. Since the early summer of 1969, my life had been filled with agony. Rather than visiting me occasionally, the arthritis became my constant companion. Worse yet, I became dependent on cortisone, which I carried with me wherever I went and had to take almost every day.

Later, I transferred to the University of California at Berkeley, believing that the climate would make a difference. The situation did not improve. I was recommended by one specialist to another, including a neurologist, an orthopedist, and a physical therapist. I lost track of the large number of blood tests and X-rays that I underwent. I could not remember how many times I had to answer the same questions about my medical history. Unable to walk to the nearest bus stop, I relied on my compassionate relatives to drive me to the different specialists.

I realized that my problem was grave, but I still kept my faith. The consultations lasted for several months without any change in therapy. The experts' final conclusion was a re-affirmation that my case was an enigma, and that it was possibly rheumatoid arthritis. My only consolation was that I did not have to worry about the costs, which must have amounted to a huge sum.

Then, disaster struck in the autumn of 1970. Within a couple of days, my knees had swollen to twice the normal size. My feet could not fit into my shoes due to swelling. I limped to the hospital and was admitted immediately. I was frightened when the doctors used a huge needle to extract the fluid from my knees. The next day, a Dr. Lee came to administer treatment. He prescribed a heavy regimen of aspirin to be taken for two weeks during which he would monitor my condition for fear of side effects.

My frustration had reached its peak. Aspirin was what I had taken when the illness first started two years previously. Now it seemed that I was back to the beginning. During those two weeks in the hospital, I was confined to bed most of the time. I was uncertain about the future and felt depressed. I had not yet written to my family about the illness, thinking that all this would be over in just a few weeks. In my darkest hours I could hear myself murmur, "Dad, I wish you were here to heal me."

My body proved that it could withstand the side effects of aspirin. I was out of the hospital in two weeks but continued on a gradually reduced dosage. Three months later, I saw Dr. Lee one last time. After finding my health restored, he proclaimed that my case was a miracle. I am forever grateful to Dr. Lee for bringing happiness back to my life. It was a pity that I could not have found him earlier.

In 1971, I graduated and returned to Hong Kong to start my career. Shortly after reuniting with my family, I received herbal treatment from my father for a couple of months. The formula he prescribed for my arthritis (see chapter 7) was aimed at eradicating the remaining "wind and dampness" trapped in my body, which according to Chinese medicine is the cause of arthritis. In addition, I have been following his advice on prevention: protect the body against sudden changes in the weather; avoid long exposures to environmental cold, wind and dampness; avoid overexertion; get enough rest; and abstain from alcohol. Since then, I have only infrequent recurrences with diminished intensity.

My experience with Western medicine was marked by suspense, frustration, endless testing and consultations, and high costs which fortunately for me, were absorbed by insurance. I wanted to know what caused my illness, but the specialists could not come to a definite conclusion. I wanted to change my habits to prevent the illness from coming back, but I was offered no advice on prevention. Had it not been for Dr. Lee, I could have wound up in a never-ending circle of consultations and drug dependency.

Chinese medical theory is rooted in a philosophy based on the nature of the universe. The theory as a whole has been largely preserved and accepted in its original context. Although it appears out of date, one can easily appreciate the wisdom of prevention and therapy accumulated over the millenia. Through my own experience, I , too, have come to appreciate the benefits of Chinese medicine, and am continually awed by its mysterious wonders.

The number and diversity of patients bearing witness lend credibility to a physician and to the medicine. The acceptability of a foreign medicine takes much more than that. Chinese medicine operates in a low-tech, low-cost, and low-profile environment. Consequently, it does not create a dramatic impression like Western medicine does. Despite constantly being refined, Chinese medical theory has largely retained its antiquity and symbolism. The preventive and therapeutic methods have become part of Chinese custom and folklore. This has created a mystique about the theory, and a barrier of understanding for people of a different culture. It also poses a communication problem for those who want to acquire or transmit the knowledge.

The major achievements of Chinese medicine lie in prevention and treatment of common illnesses. Its healing process generates few side effects and no addiction to the medicine. During the past few decades, many Chinese herbs have been analyzed in the laboratory to determine their chemical components. The published results support their therapeutic effects.

This book is organized as follows. Chapter 1 introduces the characteristics and the theory of Chinese medicine. Chapters 2 through 6 recount actual situations based on my father's diary and recollections over his sixty years of medical practice in Asia and America. In these stories we illuminate the important aspects of Chinese medicine and the circumstances under which it works. Chapter 7 presents a list of herbal prescriptions for common ailments. The prescriptions are intended as a guideline for medical practitioners who want to refine their skills in formulating herbal prescriptions. Chapter 8 discusses prevention and self-help, and highlights the health values of some popular Chinese dishes and delicacies. This chapter also explains how to make special health foods using certain raw materials and herbs.

John Fung, 1994

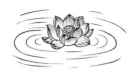

Chapter 1

An Overview Of
Traditional Chinese Medicine

The Three Branches Of
Traditional Chinese Medicine

Chinese medical theory is based on the philosophy that regards life, health, and nature as a delicate integrated system. We become ill when the equilibrium of this system is disturbed. Medicine is used to restore the balance, but that is only part of the cure. The other part lies in prevention. Through prevention, we learn more about our physcial and emotional nature in order to maintain equilibrium within ourselves. To preserve external equilibrium, we learn how to live in harmony with nature and how its cycles of change affect our health. The more we appreciate these important relationships, the better health we shall enjoy.

Traditional Chinese medicine is comprised of three branches: acupuncture, traditional orthopedics, and herbology. Acupuncture involves inserting hair-thin needles at various points on the body to heal and relieve pain. According to its theory, a system of channels carries the "vital energy" and blood throughout the human body. The channels connect the internal organs with the superficial tissues thus making the body an organic whole. Certain points on the body surface represent the places of direct connection to a particular internal organ. By inserting needles at the correct points on the body, the physician can regulate the flow of vital energy and blood to that internal organ, thereby curing the ailment originating from its source.

Traditional Chinese orthopedics is virtually unknown in the West. It specializes in healing fractured bones and dislocated joints. With fractures, the bones are set by traditional methods, then herbs are applied externally and the area is bandaged. Dislocated joints are also treated by traditional methods, followed by herbs to be applied externally or taken orally.

The third branch of Chinese medicine called herbology is comparable to internal medicine due to its broad and general coverage. The practice involves prescribing *materia medica*, or medicinal substances, found to have healing capabilities. (For the sake of simplicity, *materia medica* will hereafter be referred to as *herbs*, since a large portion of these medicinal substances are derived from plants.) The herbs are normally taken orally. Practitioners of the other two branches also prescribe herbs for their specific cures. Chinese medical history is full of accounts of distinguished physicians performing great feats in internal medicine. The most famous is probably Hua Tuo who lived circa 200 A.D. He is known to have performed major surgeries of the head and the abdomen using herbal anesthesia.

Distinct Characteristics

Chinese medicine has several distinct and practical characteristics. First, it stresses prevention. Although prevention requires practice over a long period, it guarantees better health and a lower cost.

Quite a number of Chinese herbs have preventive capabilities, and their effects are gentle on the body. Many can be used as ingredients in ordinary cooking to enrich the nutritional value as well as the taste (see chapter 8).

Another unique aspect of Chinese medicine is its diagnostic methods. Chinese physicians diagnose by observation, feel, touch, smell, and by asking questions. Unlike Western practice, there are no blood tests, cultures, X-rays, and the like, to support the diagnosis. Chinese physicians rely more on feel, observation, and communication with the patient to form a judgment about causes and about what therapy to institute. Despite such traditional methods, more often than not, the results obtained by Chinese physicians are successful.

A third area that Chinese medicine is known for is treatment aimed at strengthening the whole body to provide it with more ammunition to battle an illness. Through the ages, Chinese medicine has developed gentle but effective cures. In contrast, Western medicine isolates the cause of an illness, and applies as strong a treatment as possible, whether it be chemical, surgical, or another type of direct intervention. In many instances, the treatment is more harmful than the cure.

Chinese medical theory is based on a natural macroviewpoint while Western medicine has developed into a sophisticated mechanical and microviewpoint theory. The former stops at the organ level while the latter includes cells and even more minute structures. To account for the origin of an illness, Western medicine sees microorganisms such as viruses and bacteria as agents of disease, or pinpoints the malfunction or degeneration of a specific body part. On the other hand, Chinese medicine holds that disease arises when there is an imbalance of the environmental elements and a disharmony of the organs. Because Chinese medicine does not see below the organ level, it can neither confirm nor deny the existence of microorganisms. It only deals with the manifestations of an ailment, and offers an explanation based on the functional imbalance of the body. Since microorganisms infect every person, only those with functional imbalances fail to defend themselves.

Fundamental Principles

Chinese medical theory is characterized by symbolism and relativity, and is based on a common-sense view of nature and the cosmos. Simplicity and beauty can be found beneath the layer of myth that envelops the theory.

Yin and Yang

Yin and Yang are considered the two opposing fundamental cosmic forces responsible for all changes in the environment and life processes. Yin corresponds to things that are negative, passive, female, dark, cold, low-lying, contractive, descending, and the like, while the opposite is true for Yang. As applied to Chinese medicine, the vital organs also correspond to either Yin or Yang. For instance, the kidney is considered Yin and the heart Yang.

Yin and Yang are not absolute but relative forces. Since the universe is in equilibrium, one force cannot exist without the other. When one becomes stronger, the other weakens. When one reaches its zenith, the other is at its nadir. Hence, Yin contains the seed of Yang and vice versa. This assures that both forces stay in constant flux. The eternal cycle of night and day is the premier example of the Yin/Yang concept.

The pervasiveness of the Yin/Yang concept in Chinese thought caused it to be quickly adopted in Chinese medicine. Yin is said to control the internal, lower, and front parts of the body, and Yang the external, upper, and back parts. Yin represents the vital essence (or matter) of the body, and Yang the vital functions. For the whole body to perform properly, both must exist in the right balance. This means that a healthy body must be in internal equilibrium.

A body in stable equilibrium does not necessarily guarantee proper functioning. This is because the external environment is constantly changing, and can disturb the internal balance. An example is the sudden arrival of wind and rain. Under normal circumstances, the body is able to adjust to these changes. However, when the internal equilibrium is lacking, such conditions may cause a cold or a flare-up of arthritis, thus some type of intervention is necessary to restore the balance. For instance, in the winter when Yin dominates the environment because of coldness and fewer hours of sunshine, many elderly persons may suffer from various discomforts, such as body aches and joint pains. In such a case, the body requires a dominant Yang effect to maintain balance with the environment. Thus, herbs with Yang natures may be prescribed to relieve these discomforts.

Five Phases

Another set of concepts the Chinese employed to understand their surroundings is the Five Phases. Nature is seen to consist of five basic elements: water, wood, fire, earth, and metal. These five exist in great abundance in their natural forms. All man-made products originate from them. The elements are in constant interaction in order to maintain equilibrium. When an element becomes dominant or suppressed, the extreme conditions can be easily felt, such as in a desert (suppression of water), or near the mouth of an erupting volcano (dominance of fire).

In normal conditions, a system of support and restraint among the five elements must exist so that no one becomes dominant over the others. This system has evolved into two types of relationships, or sequences. The first is the generating sequence: water gives rise to wood by nourishing trees; wood generates fire and allows it to burn; fire reduces everything to ashes and returns them to earth; earth contains metals to be extracted; metal melts into a liquid like water. The following diagram illustrates this sequence.

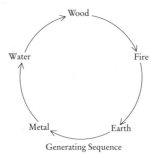

Generating Sequence

The second relationship is known as the restraining sequence: water extinguishes fire; wood (derived from trees) covers the earth and holds it together; fire melts metal; earth dams water; metal cuts wood. This sequence is shown below.

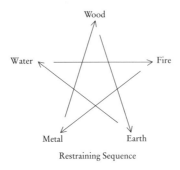

Restraining Sequence

The Five Phases as Applied to Chinese Medicine

The cardinal premise of Chinese medical theory considers the human body as a microcosm of nature.

Through the ages, the Chinese have developed numerous correspondences associated with the Five Phases, some of which have been applied in medicine. While these correspondences are abstract in nature, they have been successfully utilized to explain the origins and symptoms of diseases and to point to a direction of cure. Among the most important is the one that links the Five Phases with the five organ-pairs. The five organ-pairs are: kidney-bladder, liver-gallbladder, heart-small intestine, spleen-stomach, and lung-large intestine. These correspond, respectively, to water, wood, fire, earth, and metal. Thus, the generating and restraining sequences of the Five Phases may be applied to the organ-pairs, which, like the elements of nature, must perform as a balanced integrated unit in order to maintain normal functioning of the body. The following diagram depicts the generating and restraining sequences of the organs.

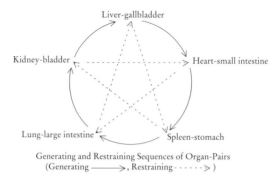

Generating and Restraining Sequences of Organ-Pairs
(Generating ———→ , Restraining - - - - - -→)

The reasoning behind the correspondence for a given organ-pair is actually quite logical, and is based on the function of the organ-pair. Starting with the kidney-bladder/water correspondence, the kidneys regulate the water content of the body. Excess water is passed to the bladder for temporary storage, then excreted as urine.

With the liver-gallbladder/wood correspondence, the liver stores vitamins and other digested food nutrients. The gallbladder stores bile. This type of function is likewise performed by the trunk of a tree which stores nutrients.

With the heart-small intestine/fire correspondence, the food essence absorbed by the small intestine is distributed throughout the body via the blood stream under the pumping action of the heart. The functions of the heart and the small intestine enable the food essence to rise and spread throughout the body. This is similar to the property of fire which rises and spreads.

With the spleen-stomach/earth correspondence, the stomach gathers and digests food. The spleen helps in the digestive process.

Both organs perform the functions of holding and containing the ingested food. This establishes the correspondence to earth which holds and contains all living and non-living things.

Finally, in the correspondence of lung-large intestine/metal, the lungs and the large intestine open the body to the outside world. The lungs react with air and absorb the Qi from it, just like metals which react with air and the moisture in it when exposed.

The correspondences associated with the Five Phases are not limited to the organs. Other parts of the body, even the emotions, can be linked to the Phases as can phenomena in nature such as the seasons. Attributes such as colors and tastes are among the other inumerable correspondences (see table below). The power of these correspondences can readily be verified by empirical evidence.

Correspondences Associated with the Five Phases

Phases	Water	Wood	Fire	Earth	Metal
Human Body					
Vital organs	Kidney	Liver	Heart	Spleen	Lung
Paired organ	Bladder	Gallbladder	S. Intestine	Stomach	L. Intestine
Sense organs	Ears	Eyes	Tongue	Mouth	Nose
Tissues	Bones	Ligaments	Arteries	Muscles	Skin & Hair
Secretions	Sexual	Tears	Sweat	Saliva	Mucus
Emotions	Fear	Anger	Joy	Pensiveness	Sadness
Conditions	Withdrawal	Arousal	Excitement	Poise	Inhibition
Awareness	Primal	Active	Transcendent	Passive	Subliminal
Tastes	Salty	Sour	Bitter	Sweet	Pungent
External elements					
Seasons	Winter	Spring	Summer	Late Summer	Autumn
Climate	Cold	Wind	Heat	Dampness	Dryness
Time	Midnight	Dawn	Noon	Late Afternoon	Dusk
Life Stage	Death	Birth	Growth	Maturity	Degeneration
Power	Consolidation	Expansion	Completion	Transition	Contraction
Directions	North	East	South	Center	West
Colors	Black	Green	Red	Yellow	White

Using the correspondence table, different empirical relationships can be observed and explained. For example, in the column under wood, the following associations can be made with the liver, gallbladder, eyes, anger, and the color green. Bile secreted by the gallbladder is green in color; when the liver malfunctions, the eyes are examined for symptoms; and finally, individuals suffering from liver conditions are prone to anger.

The restraining sequences can also be used to explain actual symptoms. Continuing with the liver/wood example, since wood restrains earth, a weak liver will fail to restrain the spleen (corresponding to earth). As a result, yellow (corresponding to earth) becomes dominant. Yellow is often the color of the sclera in the eyes of a person with a weak liver, as the eyes also correspond to wood. In addition, since the liver (wood) is restrained by the lungs (metal), sadness (metal) becomes dominant when the liver is weak. Hence, an individual suffering a liver condition can be easily overcome with sadness.

In similar fashion, the generating sequences contribute to understanding disease processes. For example, a weak liver (wood) fails to give strength to the heart (fire). This leads to a slower blood flow resulting in fatigue, and the suppression of joy (fire).

Conditions of other organs can likewise be analyzed by the Five Phase correspondences so that a more complete picture can be obtained of a disease as well as of the patient.

Qi

A sixth basic element, known as Qi (pronounced "chee"), is the vital energy on which every living thing depends. Besides circulating freely in the environment, Qi is thought to be incorporated into everything that has life including plants and animals. Plants derive their Qi from the air. An animal that eats the plants derives its Qi from the plants and the air. Similarly, humans derive their Qi from the air and food. The Qi in every living thing dissipates gradually and the rate of dissipation determines life span or longevity.

The Chinese have divided Qi into different kinds to symbolize various conditions in the external environment and in the human body. For instance, a fire type of Qi can develop internally from over-indulgence in fried or greasy foods. It can increase in intensity when the environment is hot and dry. If the fire-Qi fails to be neutralized by a cool type of Qi derived from vegetables and fruits, the individual may develop conditions such as thirst, bad breath, irritability, constipation, sleeplessness, and canker sores among others. In another example, evil-Qi arises from poor sanitation (where bacteria and viruses thrive); it can lead to serious ailment or disease and must therefore be avoided.

Qi also connotes the functional, active aspect of the body. The body itself is imbued with Qi as are the individual organs. Thus, when Qi is depleted without being replenished, disease will result.

Sources of Disease

According to Chinese medicine, there are three sources of disease: internal due to disharmony of the organs, external due to imbalance in the climate or environment, and trauma and injury. Various kinds of Qi are used to describe internal disharmonies. For example, deficiency of kidney Qi indicates that the functional aspect of the kidney is insufficient for the normal physiological activity of that organ. Treatment must therefore be aimed at replenishing the kidney Qi.

External imbalance is related to the five climatic factors of cold, wind, heat, dampness, and dryness (corresponding to water, wood, fire, earth, and metal respectively). When one or more of these environmental forces become excessive, disease may develop. For instance, a rainy spell may cause dampness to invade the bones thus giving rise to the symptoms of arthritis. In this case, herbs that dispel the dampness can be prescribed. Besides the climatic factors, there exists evil-Qi representing poor sanitation, polluted environment, or contagious diseases which may bring about illness. Herbs may then be used to strengthen the body and bolster its defense.

Trauma and injury can result in loss of blood, and according to Chinese medicine, loss of Qi. Treatment should be directed at stopping the bleeding, after which, herbs may be prescribed to replenish the blood and Qi.

In this chapter, we have briefly covered the important aspects and only some of the fundamental principles of traditional Chinese medicine. Readers who want to pursue this subject further are referred to the texts listed in the bibliography.

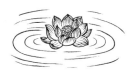

Chapter 2

Canton 1930–1937:
Where My Medical Career Began

Medical School Versus Apprenticeship

When I completed high school at eighteen, I (the senior author) wanted to work in the postal service because of the job security. At that time, the postal service in the city of Canton was controlled by France. (China had been at the mercy of the European powers since her defeat by the British in the Opium War of 1842.) I passed the written examination but failed the physical. The French doctor who examined me determined that I had a heart problem.

But, I was not concerned about my heart problem for I was more interested in finding a job. My father then advised me to study Chinese medicine. It was a respected profession even though it could not compare with the security offered by the civil service. My father had learned Chinese medicine in his spare time, and had gained experience by apprenticing with a practising herbalist. Our family had benefited from some of his prescriptions, one of which was Restore the Spleen Decoction *(gui pi tang)* which strengthens the heart and nourishes the blood. I took the prescription regularly for several months and found that it helped increase my appetite and energy.

Apprenticeship used to be the only route to becoming a practitioner of Chinese medicine. This was changing with the establishment of medical schools in some major cities. The push for a structured program in Chinese medicine was the result of a broad range of modernization policies initiated by the government and some private organizations.

The quest for modernization did not happen by chance. The awakening of China to external threats began when the Chinese experienced defeat in the Opium War at the hands of the powerful British who possessed warships with the latest military technology of the Industrial Revolution. The awakening quickly turned into great humiliation as other European powers such as France, Germany, and Russia moved in. By 1900, all the major coastal cities were carved up into sectors where foreigners lived and conducted business under the protection of their own laws and troops. These special privileges were known as extraterritorial concessions. They were in fact outright occupations by force that were legalized by treaties. Each of those treaties was signed after an incident of failed Chinese resistance against the intruders.

The Japanese later entered the scene. They demonstrated their military strength by defeating the Russian Baltic Fleet to take over the Russian sectors in northeast China. At that time, Japan was the only country in the Far East to have successfully modernized. Japan later became the fiercest and most brutal of all aggressors against China. For the Chinese, World War II did not begin in September 1939 when German troops invaded Poland. It began earlier, in July 1937, when Japan initiated a massive military campaign on the Chinese mainland. By 1942, shortly after Pearl Harbor, half of the Japanese army was already stationed on Chinese soil, with a total of six million troops occupying the entire coastal region. The Japanese troops had liquidated all the European sectors and taken control of all European interests in China.

In August 1945, the Japanese surrender and withdrawal from China ended more than one hundred years of foreign tyranny. The period from 1842 up to the end of World War II is to me the darkest and saddest part of Chinese history. Frankly, I did not think that China could survive as a nation with foreign powers controlling her most important territories and interests.

In addition to the external threats to her sovereignty, China's internal struggle for modernization was protracted. In 1911, China became a republic after the overthrow of the decadent Qing dynasty. The revolution of 1911 could not save China. The country was immediately thrown into chaos when regional warlords asserted their power. The central government of the Nationalist Party ruled in name only. The formation of the Communist Party several years later split the country even further. The conflict between the two major parties later erupted into a civil war culminating in the Communist victory in October 1949. I can only describe with tears the sufferings of the Chinese people during those years when wars, foreign aggression, government corruption, political chaos, economic depression, and hyper-inflation all converged at the same time.

In the quest for modernization, Chinese medicine almost became a casualty. Many Chinese students went to Europe and Japan to study the new technologies and political systems. Upon return, they were anxious to reform anything traditional which was thought to hamper Chinese progress. In 1929, a group of returning medical graduates from Japan recommended legislation to abolish Chinese medicine. The proposal was vigorously rejected at a national medical assembly later that year. The outrageous proposal was aimed at destroying a national heritage that had worked for so many centuries. Fortunately, the pragmatists gained the upper hand over the zealots. In 1933, the government estab-

lished the Central Chinese Hospital for the systemization and pro-
motion of Chinese medicine. This encouraged the establishment
of more medical schools all over the country. As a consequence,
Chinese medicine could be studied in a structured academic program rather than through apprenticeship.

In 1930, I passed the entrance examination and was admitted
to the Canton College of Chinese Medicine. The College was
financed by a group of physicians and herb merchants. It operated a four-story hospital where all new graduates interned for one
year. There was also an herb farm on one corner of the campus.
The students learned how herbs were cultivated and processed.
The course work lasted four years and included all branches of
Chinese medicine. I chose to specialize in herbology.

The heavy emphasis on practical experience resulted in the students spending most of their time in the hospital and on the herb
farm. In the hospital, we studied how our professors diagnosed
and applied therapy. We observed the healing effects of herbs on
the patients and discovered that most herbs have multiple and overlapping effects. We also learned how to produce special healing
effects by combining the herbs in various proportions. The most
difficult skill to master was controlling the effects of all the herbs
in a single prescription because of the number of combinations
possible. Other students and I would perform experiments with
herbs on one another. Through such experiments, I learned the
fine details about the effects of herbs on different people under
various conditions. This practical experience constituted the most
precious part of my medical education.

My training did not stop after graduation. Knowledge is gained
mostly through real-life experimentation and empirical evidence.
In Chinese medicine, prescriptions do not follow a fixed pattern
guided by an exact theory or procedure. I constantly refined my
knowledge and skills through trial and error with many patients.
Through the years, I gained a great deal of insight which increased

my success. Most of my patients were healed after two consultations. My own skills notwithstanding, I have relied on the faith of my patients to allow me to perfect a cure. I have also relied on the herbs which produce a gradual effect so that I can adjust ensuing prescriptions accordingly.

During my school years, Western medicine had greatly impressed the intelligentsia with its new discoveries. To keep students up to date, our course work also included the latest developments in Western medicine. We were fascinated by the anatomy of the human body as illustrated in the reading materials. However, dissection was not performed in our school because the human body was considered sacred in Chinese society. There were also strong objections against dissecting the body solely for studying the various parts. More importantly, Chinese medicine views the human body as a natural whole and does not impose the necessity of learning the minute details of its parts.

Private Practice Interrupted By War

In 1935, after one year of internship, I set up my own private practice in Canton. I obtained a license from the city health department. It cost fifteen Chinese dollars. During that time, the average monthly salary was around forty dollars and rent was about fifteen dollars. I charged forty cents per consultation. The herbs which patients would buy with my prescription from an herb store nearby cost about the same. Many patients could not afford the payment, and in such cases, I simply waived the fees. Others willingly paid more to show their appreciation, in which case, I proudly accepted.

My office measured about fifty feet by ten feet. A small enclosure was set up at one end for conducting physical examinations and for private discussions. Most consultations were done at my desk outside the enclosure where I performed regular diagnostic routines. There was no need for a nurse or assistant. I sat facing the entrance so that I knew how many patients there were as they came in and sat down to await their turns on a row of seats arranged by the wall. On the opposite side, there was a couch for patients too weak to sit up. This office arrangement was typical of the simple, open, and personalized approach of this profession. Sitting facing the entrance also gave me an opportunity to assess the conditions of my patients through their postures as they approached my desk.

It was customary for a physician to display in the office the gifts presented by appreciative patients. In the beginning, I only had a few that were given by some friends to make my office look nicer. As time went by, I accumulated many more from my patients. The gifts usually consisted of frames to be hung on the wall. The most popular was a set of Chinese calligraphy which translated meant the reincarnation of Hua Tuo, the legendary Chinese physician of the second century.

The Japanese aggression quickly spread southward. In December 1937, the capital city of Nanking fell. Chinese resistance had resorted to guerrilla warfare. The central government began its retreat to the hinterland. The people were horrified to learn about the large-scale massacres and rapes committed by Japanese troops in Nanking. The city of Canton was now subject to daily bombardment by the Japanese air force. There was little doubt that Canton would soon fall. The population either had to flee inland, or to the British colony of Hong Kong ninety miles away where British troops might be able to deter the Japanese onslaught. I left my medical practice and sought shelter in Hong Kong with the rest of the family.

Alcohol Almost Destroys My Best Friend

Alcohol is a human invention for adding some spice to life. Limited and conscientious consumption can bring about appetite enhancement and better blood circulation. However, too much can only do harm.

One hot summer night in Canton, my best friend Mok and I, and a couple of other friends went to enjoy the cool breezes on the water of Lychee Bay. This was a favorite pastime for ordinary citizens in the city. There were plenty of boats for hire, ranging from small two-seaters to large ones for holding parties. After sunset, the Bay was dotted with these boats bearing lanterns. The calm water, the cool breeze, and the full moon together made a pleasant and romantic atmosphere. Occasionally, food peddlers on boats passed by selling fruits, beverages, fried clams, noodles, and seafood porridge. If one was in the mood for music, a boat carrying a band of musicians was waiting to serenade and play one's favorite tunes. For those who wanted to stay close to shore, they could paddle along the embankment lined with lychee trees whose fruits were ripe for picking in the summer. We ate, drank, talked, and laughed until nearly 3 A.M. Mok was more than half-drunk. We walked back with him to his house to ensure his safety.

The next day Mok came to my office. He had a slight fever but looked very tired. The lower part of his body was swollen. He felt pain when urinating. Mok used to have some minor kidney problems. He told me that the night before, he took a cold shower before going to bed, and was awakened later because he felt cold. I thought that he had caught a cold, which was aggravated by too much alcohol. My immediate concern was to reduce the swelling and the fever. I gave him a prescription to strengthen the kidneys and clear the water from his body. It worked as expected initially. However, he came back after three days in worse condition. This time, his face and eyes were swollen, and he had no appetite.

I consulted my former teacher, Professor Chang. After examining Mok, he concluded that it was a case of alcohol poisoning of the kidneys. The water accumulated in the body was due to malfunction of the kidneys. A weak kidney would fail to restrain

the heart, according to Chinese medicine, and would also lead to
a weak liver.

Mok's case could easily develop into heart and liver problems if it were not treated immediately. Professor Chang wrote a
prescription containing cinnamon twig *(gui zhi)*, codonopsis *(dang
shen)*, eucommia *(du zhong)*, cornus *(shan zhu yu)*, and ginger
(gan jiang) as the main ingredients. The formula was aimed at neutralizing the alcohol poisoning and restoring the Yin-Yang balance
of the kidneys. The herbs produced a great deal of urination and
watery stools for several days. Mok gradually recovered although
it took almost a month. Later, Mok recalled how bad he felt, and
had actually thought that he would die. From this experience, I
learned about the great damage that excessive alcohol can render,
even to an occasional drinker, although Mok's case was exceptional
due to kidney complications.

A White Lie Prevents The Breakup Of A Family

One late afternoon just as I was about to end my work day, a couple and an elderly woman came into the office. They seemed to
have been arguing heatedly. The younger woman sat down, wip-
ing her eyes with a handkerchief. The man was visibly angry. He
and the elderly woman asked if I knew about the "white flower
disease." I did not. However, since Chinese medicine is so rich in
symbolism, the disease might well be a common one which I had
learned under a different name. Sensing that this might be a con-
fidential matter, I invited the man and the elderly woman into the
enclosure to better understand the situation.

I learned that it was a family problem I had to resolve. The couple were newlyweds. The elderly woman was the man's mother.
After the honeymoon, the husband discovered that the wife was
not a virgin because he did not see any blood immediately after the
first sexual intercourse. The man felt betrayed. It is a long-held Chinese tradition that the woman is supposed to keep her virginity to

demonstrate good faith to the man she is to marry. The husband was also frustrated because his wife refused to admit or deny anything. He and his mother wanted me to confirm that the wife indeed had the "white flower disease," which as they understood, would explain the absence of blood. What should I do? I could turn them away and say that this was not my specialty. However, I realized that a physician has a special social responsibility in traditional Chinese society.

I asked them to leave the enclosure so that I could invite the younger woman in for a private talk. The wife was very frank. She admitted that her first marriage had ended with the death of her husband in another province some four years ago. However, she did not have the courage to tell this to her second husband. She wanted me to keep the secret and to persuade the husband to keep her in the family. She also pledged that she would be faithful to the second husband whom she loved dearly.

My medical duty suddenly took on the new dimension as arbitrator. I had just received the trust and faith bestowed to the medical profession by a troubled family. Nobody in this family knew me previously. They trusted me because herbalists were very respected in our community. My compelling sense of duty was to save this family from a potential breakup. I must disregard prevailing traditions and medical technicalities. The answer to this problem was already provided by the husband. All I needed to do was to confirm it although I doubted very much that such a disease existed.

I talked to both parties again separately. I pointed out the possible existence of the "white flower disease" which might invalidate the proof of a female's virginity. But I also emphasized that the most important thing for a family is to love and care for each other despite doubts and difficulties. Both parties accepted my points readily. They agreed that they should put this matter behind them and direct their energies toward building a happy family. The husband asked how much he owed me. I did not feel I should charge them any fee. However, he paid one Chinese dollar and insisted that I should accept it.

A few months later, the mother of the husband stopped by and happily reported that her daughter-in-law was pregnant. Shortly before leaving Canton for Hong Kong, I learned with great distress that the street on which they lived had been decimated by bombs. I prayed that they had escaped the ravages of war, but thereafter I never had any news of them.

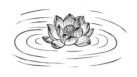

Chapter 3

Hong Kong 1938–1939: Temporary Shelter From War

Resident Physician and Private Practice

My entire family fled to the British colony of Hong Kong in January 1938. In October that year, Canton fell. A contingent of British forces guarding Hong Kong was now facing the Japanese army within binocular's distance on the Chinese mainland. Some kinds of foodstuff had to be rationed in Hong Kong. Electricity was cut most of the nights to protect the city from aerial bombardment. This tense standoff continued into December 1941 when Japan attacked Pearl Harbor and unleashed an all-out offensive against the European forces stationed in Asia. Hong Kong fell in December 1941, so did other major cities in Southeast Asia.

Having been dislocated from Canton, I had to start my private practice all over again in Hong Kong. I set up my home office in Kowloon District in 1938. Most of my patients could not pay their fees due to the depressed economy. My private practice became a free clinic for the poor. I therefore joined the Tung Wah Group of Hospitals as a resident physician. This enabled me to make a living and maintain my private practice in the evenings and on the weekends.

Hemorrhoid Is A Longtime Discomfort

Hemorrhoid is an inflamed tissue that develops close to the anus. Many adults are affected by hemorrhoids. The common causes include anal infection, straining during bowel movements, and intra-abdominal pressure resulting from pregnancy. Minor cases produce itching and slight bleeding; more serious ones may require surgery to remove the hemorrhoid.

Mr. Lau had had a mild hemorrhoid for a long time. He used to treat it externally with Chinese herbs. There were several standard ones available at the herb store. The medicine existed in either powder or paste form which could be applied to the inflammation. Usually, such remedies produced a soothing and gradual healing effect. However, the hemorrhoid often developed again in the same location after a short period of relief. So Lau came and asked me for a permanent cure.

I discovered that Lau did not pay attention to personal hygiene. He did not bathe regularly, especially during winter. He liked barbecued and peppery foods which invariably provoked heat in the body. An increase in heat would thus cause inflammation of the hemorroidal tissue. Lau described himself as a carnivore for he disliked vegetables. The constipation that he often had attested to his unbalanced diet. Lau complained that when the hemorrhoid was just starting to heal, the straining during bowel movements would open the old wound and cause bleeding again. I pointed out to Lau that the answers to a permanent cure lay in changing his old habits.

Meanwhile, I prescribed some herbs that would reduce the inflammation by controlling the heat in the body. A gentle laxative was included to soften the stool. Lau took the prescription regularly for more than two months and gradually changed his dietary and hygiene habits. The hemorrhoid showed signs of healing. I cautioned Lau that hemorrhoids do not go away easily and that it would take a long time for a permanent cure.

Some Interesting Facets Of Superstition

Because there were many practitioners of traditional medicine, a patient who wanted to consult an herbalist had difficulty in deciding whom to go to. Usually, patients based their selection on personal experience, word of mouth, or they just went to the physician in the neighborhood. Quite a few patients employed other interesting methods of selection.

The Buddhist temple used to be a popular place to seek help. Believers could ask for divine advice in locating the best physician by kneeling in front of the altar and talking to the gods. Then they would pick up a cylindrical container which held a few dozen wooden sticks with a number carved on each, and shake the container until one stick came out. The number on the chosen stick would point to a piece of printed advice which the believer could ask a priest or a specialist at the temple to explain.

The advice usually indicated in which direction the physician lived, how many strokes there were in the Chinese character of the physician's surname, or whether the surname character contained certain desired parts. Indeed many of my own patients asked me if I lived in the east relative to their residences, and some were happy to find me because the character of my surname contained two strokes on the left, which meant water, often found to be desirable.

While some express condescension toward such patients for their superstitious beliefs, I reserve judgment in this regard. Knowledge is constantly expanding. Many theories or explanations we hold today as reasonable are waiting to be disproved or overthrown in the future. The human mind has a limited capacity for understanding everything surrounding us. Some things we shall never be able to find a definite answer for; many others will unfold as time goes on and new knowledge is acquired.

Faith and belief are often founded on culture and tradition. They also vary according to the knowledge that an individual possesses at a given time. For example, people in ancient times—even some in our own time—believe that lightning and thunder were an expression of God's anger. Now that we know the cause of lightning and thunder, we brand this ancient belief as superstition. To cite a modern example, many people believe that technology is the solution to all of our problems. Some even believe that computers will save the world. I would not be surprised if some popular beliefs we hold today were to be considered preposterous a few years from now. In the final analysis, it should matter very little whether we will be proven right or wrong. From a practical standpoint, we need something to believe in to keep us moving forward.

A Ticket To Vietnam

The Tung Wah Group of Hospitals in Hong Kong had connections with other hospitals established by overseas Chinese living in Southeast Asia. I had learned that the Cantonese Hospital in the city of Cholon in Vietnam wanted to hire two physicians. For many years, Southeast Asia had been a favorite place for Chinese immigrants. Furthermore, the small island of Hong Kong could not possibly survive should the Japanese decide to attack it. Then where should I seek refuge? So I applied for the job amid 113 other applicants. Candidate selection was administered by the Tung Wah Hospital.

The first written examination eliminated the great majority of applicants. I was among the six finalists who went for the practical examination held at Tung Wah Hospital. We were taken to a convalescence room where four patients were staying. We were given an hour and a half to diagnose and write a prescription for each patient. The only restriction was that we could not ask the patients any questions. This of course did not correspond to the real-life situation, but I guessed that the examiners wanted to see how experienced we were with respect to other methods of diagnosis.

I carefully observed, felt, touched, smelled, and read the pulse of each of the patients. The first one was a middle-aged male suffering from high blood pressure and recovering from a liver disease. The second was a younger woman whose menstrual problems had weakened her. The third was an elderly woman suffering from a sudden flare-up of arthritis. The fourth was a small boy recovering from diarrhea. I explained in detail my diagnoses, and wrote down the prescriptions according to my judgments regarding these four cases.

Two months later, the Tung Wah Hospital informed me that I had been selected. I had to assume duty as soon as possible. I left Hong Kong on Christmas eve in 1939 with Dr. Leung who was the other applicant selected. There we were, two bachelors leaving war-torn China to seek a better future in Vietnam. It had never occurred to us that we would be staying there for the greater part of our careers. We left our families behind hoping that the war would soon be over, and that we would come back to resume our private practices.

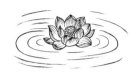

Chapter 4

Saigon 1939–1969:
Home Away From Home

The Chinese Settlers In Southeast Asia

All the major cities of Southeast Asia have large Chinese populations, over twenty million in total. A significant portion can trace their origins to the coastal provinces of southern China. A great majority have settled in Southeast Asia for generations. Through intermarriage with the native population, the Chinese settlers have been assimilated into the local communities. In fact, most have adopted native surnames and become citizens of the countries they live in. Vietnam and Singapore are two exceptions where the Chinese settlers maintain a more distinct identity.

As in the rest of Southeast Asia, Chinese settlers in Vietnam established various businesses and industries. Consequently, they controlled a significant part of the local economy. This led to social conflicts which resulted in legislation designed to enhance the economic power of the natives. In Vietnam, relations between Chinese settlers and natives were more harmonious compared to other countries in the region.

When I arrived in Saigon in late 1939, I was surprised by the sprawling Chinatown of Cholon whose population was around two million. Downtown Cholon was not much different from Canton for it was easily immersed in Chinese culture and tradition. Vietnam was part of French Indochina then. It was officially a territory of the French Union. The French had established their seat of government in the twin cities of Saigon-Cholon to administer the southern part of the country.

My long thirty-year stay in Vietnam left me with many happy as well as sad memories. The happy ones are related to my success in private practice, my marriage to Jing and the raising of our four children, and to many friends with whom I remain in contact today. The sad memories include my witnessing the difficult birth of the Republic of South Vietnam, the protracted war with the Vietcong, the failure of the massive American intervention, and the degeneration of the Republic leading to its eventual downfall in 1975.

The Chinese Slave Workers

Shortly after the Pearl Harbor attack, Japanese troops swept into Saigon. One day, a jeep and three trucks arrived at the front entrance of the Cantonese Hospital. A Japanese officer with a local interpreter came in and asked to see a resident physician. I happened to be on duty that day. Through the interpreter, I learned that they wanted us to treat one hundred and sixty people who were already being off-loaded from the trucks. I was given a list of their names and asked to sign at the bottom. The interpreter then delivered a short speech in Cantonese to the sick people and gave a stern warning that they would be shot if they tried to escape.

After the officer left, I immediately ordered these people to be housed in two halls of the hospital. We did not have enough beds for this sudden influx of patients and had to make do with mattresses on the floor. These people were male captives, mostly from Canton. They were mainly suffering from malnutrition, dysentery, and fever. The resources of the hospital were stretched to the limit for one entire week as we attended to them.

In my spare time, I managed to talk to the majority of these captives. A Mr. Kwan told me that he and his wife were captured from a street in Canton during the Japanese occupation. A day later, together with other captives, they were led to a Japanese transport ship and set sail. After reaching Saigon, he was put in a military camp as a slave worker. He had no idea where his wife was. I asked the captives to write down the names and addresses of their relatives so that the hospital might be able to contact them later.

The Japanese officer came back after a week when he learned that the men had recovered. My tears streamed down as I watched my countrymen return involuntarily to their cruel captors. I cursed myself for not being able to do anything more than provide cure and comfort.

My New Practice In Cholon

When World War II ended in August 1945, I thought about whether to return to Canton to resume my private practice. I was discouraged to learn that the civil war in China had flared up again between the Communists and the Nationalists. Furthermore, I had already established a solid reputation with the patients during my five years as a resident physician. The owner of an herb firm in Cholon asked if I wanted to join him as a partner. I agreed after several days of discussions.

The arrangement was typical: the herb shop provided an in-house office for the physician whose reputation could attract more patients thus enhancing its business, and the physician wanted an in-house office to make it more convenient for the patients to obtain herbs after consultation. The consultation fees would be pocketed by the physician, while the charges for the herbs would go to the shop owner. The name of this herb shop was "hundred complete shop," implying that we had everything the patients needed.

Our business picked up gradually. The clientele grew to include many Vietnamese who used Chinese medicine, and as a result, my Vietnamese improved. A couple of years later, Kwui, the shop owner, ran into some financial difficulties. I invested my savings in the herb store and became co-owner with Kwui. An employee of the herb shop suggested that I devote one afternoon a week to providing free consultations. So I did on every Wednesday afternoon. The kindness and goodwill of the free consultations generated a high volume of business for the herb store. This encouraged many other practitioners to follow suit. We might have sacrificed some, but the benefits to society and ourselves were beyond measure.

Running an herb shop while maintaining my medical duties quickly taxed my energy to the limits. I therefore concentrated on making the purchasing decisions and left the accounting, personnel, and inventory management to Kwui. Nearly all the herbs were imported from China via Hong Kong. The salesmen representing different import houses came to our shop twice a week. They brought samples, explained the healing effects, and gave us price quotations. In between consultations, I found time to inspect and taste the samples, decide how much we needed, and negotiate the final price. Through this I acquired a first-hand knowledge of herbs and their different grades. I also learned about the conditions that affected the supply of herbs. I was impressed by the fact that although China was going through a difficult period, its export of herbs was relatively stable. We had only encountered infrequent shortages for a few kinds of herbs.

My private practice and herb business prospered. I developed many friendships and business associates. My patients kept referring their acquaintances to me. I learned through experience that the key to successful practice is to empathize with, and care for my patients and their families. In return they placed their faith and trust in me. The initial patient-doctor relationships developed naturally into lasting friendships. It is my conviction that a successful medical practice requires the three ingredients of care, faith, and trust which must exist between the physician and the patient.

I realized that I was a most fortunate person when I met Jing around 1944. Love for Cantonese opera brought us together. Our common interest also gave me a good excuse to visit her every night at her mother's house. I conveyed my feelings for her through all the love songs I could possibly find in Cantonese music. We were married a year later. Jing's family had settled in Vietnam at about the same time as I did. Her mother was a midwife and operated her own business next door. We later had four wonderful children. In the late 1950s, we became naturalized citizens of South Vietnam, and made Cholon our home away from home.

Fever And Diarrhea: Children's Common Ailments

Fever accompanied by diarrhea was a common ailment among children in Cholon. There were many reasons. First, the hot weather promoted the multiplication of insects and the spread of disease. Second, food peddlers abounded, and attracted children with pocket money to spend. Much of the food sold was easily contaminated by flies and other insects. Third, frequent celebration of traditional and religious festivals involved feasting, and children often became sick from too much eating. Fourth, small children were often given powdered or canned milk rather than being breast fed. Refrigerators were not common household items at that time, so children were sometimes given milk that had gone bad in the hot weather.

One case that I recall was the four-year-old son of a Mr. and Mrs. Pan. The boy was suffering from fever and diarrhea, and had been treated by another physician with no improvement. The diarrhea occurred almost every two hours with the passing of watery stools. The boy looked very weak because most of what he ate could not be retained. The diarrhea and occasional vomiting also complicated the treatment procedure as the prescription had to be taken orally and might not be absorbed by the digestive system.

Something had to be done to strengthen the child and stop the diarrhea. I told the parents to feed the boy at hourly intervals with small quantities of thin rice soup with some sugar added. The soup with no meat and oil could thus be easily absorbed by the digestive system. After several feedings, the boy seemed to be gaining strength. Then a small dosage of prescription was given to stop the diarrhea and cool the fever. The hourly feeding continued for two days, followed by more normal feeding with some fish and vegetables added. The prescription was given three times a day. Within a week the boy was restored to health.

After the boy's recovery, his grandparents invited me to their home for tea. I learned that their family had a large raw material import and export business. The grandfather also operated a local Chinese newspaper. He later published some good comments about my healing results. Such recommendations by an influential family like the Pans boosted my credibility. Later, I became their family doctor and the boy became my godson as an expression of gratitude from his parents.

My Longest Day in a Flu Season

Influenza is a contagious disease that strikes in population centers around the world. In San Francisco, we occasionally experience a particularly severe flu season. But the flu that we see in America cannot compare with what I saw in Vietnam with regard to intensity, frequency, and spread.

During my thirty years of practice in the Saigon-Cholon area, the flu struck one or two times a year. The major factor was poor sanitation, typical of a developing country. The occurrence of the flu followed the pattern of seasonal changes, appearing usually in the spring when growth began. A person who caught the flu developed a high fever in a matter of hours. Other symptoms included headache, joint pain, coughing, runny nose, phlegm, and an alternating sensation of heat and chills. After treatment, the flu receded swiftly in a couple of days. The flu epidemic in the city usually lasted about three weeks. There were few fatalities as a direct result of the flu.

One day in March of 1960 at the height of the flu season, I woke up at 5 A.M. and hurried through my morning routine. I stopped by the bedside of my youngest daughter to make sure that her fever was under control. There was already a commotion at the door. Some patients had arrived and were waiting outside. One of the three servants in the household rushed to the door and told them to wait quietly, for the doctor was not ready yet. My two teenage sons were up by this time. They went outside to count the patients and kept them in line. Around 6 A.M., one son reported that there were already over twenty patients outside. I told him to let them in. The patients spilled over into our living room next to my home office, and thus began my longest day.

The average consultation lasted for ten minutes. The charge was fifteen Vietnamese piastres as compared with the monthly wage of seven hundred piastres for a live-in servant. For each patient, I prescribed herbs for one day's use. When the patient came back the next day, I would be able to see the effects of the herbs and the condition of the patient. This would allow me to perfect the second prescription and finalize the cure. When treating the flu, the goal is to reduce the fever, restore the balance of the body functions disrupted by the flu, to relax the body, and finally to strengthen the body to enable a swift recovery.

At 7 A.M., one of our maids accompanied three of our four children to school. My wife carried on the job of attending to the waiting patients. The living room was still crowded. At 8:00 A.M., an employee at the herb store came and informed me that many patients were waiting there. My wife asked the latecomers to go to the herb store which was only two blocks away.

Shortly before 9 A.M., I finished with the last patient at home. I went back to check on our youngest one who was now up and playing in bed. I wrote a prescription and told my wife that this should be the last one to finish off her fever. Then the cook told me that she might have caught the flu, too. I prescribed some herbs which would strengthen her body to guard against the flu. I grabbed the newspaper and left for the herb store. A "cyclo" was waiting at the door. It was a tricycle with a covered passenger seat at the front. I usually took a cyclo to the herb store so that I could spend a few quiet moments browsing the newspaper before my day began. On my way out the door, a maid was cleaning the living room. My wife was collecting the cash in the drawer to deposit in the bank.

I started working immediately after arriving at the herb store. The five employees were already busily packaging the herbs for patients who saw me earlier at home. The morning went by quickly. I took a one-hour lunch break at one of the many restaurants nearby. The wife of the restaurant owner came to my table and asked for a prescription, as did a couple of her employees. After lunch, I went back to the herb store to face the long line again. My office hour ended at 6 P.M. By that time, everyone at the store was completely exhausted. One employee had come down with a fever, all the others needed some strengthening herbs, including myself.

I took the same pedicab home to join my family. Some patients were already waiting in the living room. They had been diverted there by the herb store employees shortly before the end of my office hour. I spent another hour treating patients at home. Then came dinner. I was happy to see our youngest one at the table. Her fever was gone. For the next few days, we only gave her rice gruel cooked with some fish, minced beef or pork, and some steamed vegetables on the side. She also had some orange, pear, or banana.

This light but balanced diet helped her recover. A regular diet during the recovery period would only invite the fever back, a common occurrence in small children.

After dinner, before another patient could catch me, my wife and I dashed off to the Cantonese Expatriate Association a few blocks away. We frequented this club for recreation. Among their many activities, I enjoyed singing Cantonese opera while being accompanied by a group of amateur instrumentalists. As expected, some friends came to me and requested prescriptions. Some people struck by the flu whom I did not know also interrupted my evening. A few of them were surprised at my sudden burst of temper for which I felt sorry afterward. The activities at the club ended around 10:30. Then we went out for a noodle snack, and returned home around 11:30, only to find yet more patients waiting to see me. Finally at midnight, after the last patient had left, I was able to relax in tranquility and replenish my energy for another grueling day.

Heat In The Body: A Source Of Many Discomforts

The climate of Southeast Asia is characterized by heat and humidity for most of the year. The heat and humidity permeate into the human body and are known in Chinese medicine as the pathogenic factors of Heat and Dampness. In this type of climate, salty and peppery foods are desirable because they stimulate the appetite which is dulled by the hot weather. Peppery food dispels the Dampness in the body. However, the hotness of pepper increases the Heat. The excess heat is not an illness but is enough to cause many kinds of discomfort. Conditions commonly seen include canker sores, constipation, hemorrhoid itching, nose bleeds, sleeplessness, and emotional irritation. To resolve these conditions, people drink iced water and eat juicy fruits, especially watermelon. However, certain kinds of tropical fruit increase both Heat and

Dampness in the body. One such fruit is durian. I used to like it but hate the discomfort it creates. Other such fruits are pineapple and coconut which tend to promote Dampness.

Excess Heat in the body is a common condition not limited to tropical countries. In America, people like to eat barbecued and deep-fried foods, roasted nuts, potato chips, and the like. These are cooked or processed in direct contact with fire and oil, a process that incorporates another pathogenic factor, Fire, into the food. After being absorbed into the body, Fire immediately causes thirst. To quench the thirst, beer or some type of iced beverage is desired. However, Heat in the body cannot be dispelled easily just by drinking cold beverages. Eating juicy fruits such as watermelon, pear, orange, or grapefruit over a period of several days proves to be the best method. To reduce the absorption of Fire into the body, steam cooking should be employed since it is water that comes into direct contact with the food thus weakening the Fire. It should be mentioned that drinking coffee also promotes Heat because coffee beans are processed by roasting which allows Fire to be incorporated into the beans.

Sometimes excess Heat can persist such that a person has to seek treatment. Mr. Chen was a bellboy in a hotel near my residence in Cholon. One evening he came by and told me that he could not swallow any food due to pain near the throat. He did not appear ill and had no temperature when I felt his forehead. However, I could see that his eyes were red, his lips were swollen and red, and I could smell his bad breath. His pulse was normal, showing no signs of organ malfunction. After questioning him about the food he ate for the past week, I concluded that he had excess heat in the body. I inspected the inside of his mouth and saw some canker sores. His tongue had a thick yellow fur which confirmed his complaint about not being able to taste certain foods. His uvula was swollen and there was a red blister on it. When I touched it, he indicated that it was the same pain he experienced when trying to swallow food.

I punctured the blister with an acupuncture needle to release the blood. Then I gave him a cup of cold water to drink. The pain was gone immediately. I explained to him that his was an extreme case of excess heat. I advised him that he should balance the spicy food he ate with lots of vegetables and fruits. I also gave him a prescription consisting of American ginseng *(xi yang shen)*, glehnia *(sha shen)*, ophiopogon *(mai men dong)*, and licorice *(gan cao)*, which would clear the Heat and moisten the throat.

Heat discomfort has long bred a significant consumer industry in China and Southeast Asia. In Canton, the "cool tea" shops on many busy streets offered cups of black tea at a low price. The tea was made from a standard formula of twenty-four kinds of herbs that clear excess Heat. In Saigon, the streets were lined with stands selling iced sugarcane juice and other fruit juices.

In Hong Kong, resourceful entrepreneurs of "cool tea" shops set up jukeboxes, television sets, and comfortable chairs. Others offered hot and tasty fried bean curd and curried fried squid which would inevitably increase the Heat of the body. Thus, customers intending to "cool off" were tempted to order the tasty hot stuff. This would of course increase the Heat, hence driving them to consume more "cool tea." This was certainly a devious way to attract business.

Apart from vegetables and fruits which can be used to neutralize Heat, I would like to recommend the popular Chinese delicacy of dried green beans and sliced kelp. These two ingredients are available in most oriental food markets. The delicacy is prepared by boiling together (with a bit of rice if preferred) in water for several hours to make a nutritious broth. Adding sugar makes a tasty snack. Many people like to add crushed ice to make a cold drink. Apart from this delicacy, water chestnuts are also effective in neutralizing Heat. After peeling the skin, these can be eaten raw, or chopped into small pieces to be cooked with other vegetables.

Herbs To Maintain Body Equilibrium

Mrs. Wong was one of many patients who consulted me regularly for a "tune up" prescription. Her physical condition was very
susceptible to weather changes. When the rainy season came, she
experienced fatigue and joint pain. When the weather turned cooler, she had to wear more clothing than usual to suppress the sudden bursts of chill originating within the body. During this time,
she was also afflicted by paleness and lack of energy. However, all
these routinely disappeared when the hot season came around.

Cold- and rainy-season discomfort are common among many
people over the age of forty. These conditioins are caused by an
imbalance of body functions brought about by changes in the
weather. The symptoms vary from person to person. The common element is that the symptoms will later disappear when the
cold or rainy season passes.

According to Chinese medical theory, a person can be catego-
rized as a Yin or Yang type. In the above case, Mrs. Wong belongs
to the Yin type. This means her body tends to have a Yin dominance. Yin has the characteristics of dampness, coldness, low-lying,
and inactivity. Thus, a Yin-type person will feel uncomfortable
when Yin dominates the external environment, such as during
rainy or cold weather, which throws the body functions off balance, resulting in all kinds of discomfort. To resolve this, the body
must slowly adjust to a new equilibrium with the external environment. This is where Chinese herbs come in. By taking herbs,
the body can quickly find a new equilibrium. In Mrs. Wong's case,
she needed a Yang-dominant prescription to "warm up" the body
to compensate for the influences of the Yin-dominant environment.

In contrast to a Yin-type person, a Yang-type individual will
feel more comfortable in cooler weather. In the hot season, the
conditions that affect a Yang-type person coincide more or less
with those caused by Heat as described. Heat in the body seldom

requires herbs for relief. The easiest way to dispel Heat is to eat juicy fruits and drink a lot of water.

Most young people are of the Yang-type as evidenced by their high energy and activeness during the cold seasons. As a person ages, the Yang in the body slowly loses its dominance over the Yin. Consequently, many of the older population are of the Yin-type, and show less affinity for cold weather. This is evidenced by the settlement of American retirees in the warmer, sun-belt states.

Besides the human body, all signs in the physical world indicate that Yin tends to dominate Yang in the long term. Fire, which symbolizes Yang, will eventually burn itself out after consuming everything on land. But water, which symbolizes Yin, is able to extinguish fire. Moreover, the great abundance of water on this planet will enable it to immerse all continents as the oceans comprise three-quarters of the earth's surface.

The Three Abundances That Cure

The residents of Cholon were accustomed to living along with what I liked to call the three "domestic wildlife": the lizard, the bat, and the gecko. They were nocturnal inhabitants of Vietnamese cities as well as of the countryside. Lizards and bats were uninvited cotenants of every home. Although geckos were seldom seen in the home, their "kap kerr" sound indicated their presence in the surroundings.

When darkness set in, the lizards came out from the attic and ruled the ceiling. They were a special type, three to four inches long, yellowish grey, with four short legs, and a tail. Defying gravity, they rested, walked, or ran belly-side-up on the ceiling. Many insects such as moths, flies, mosquitos, and spiders, liked to gather around the ceiling fluorescent lights. The lizards gingerly approached and caught them with their tongues. The walls or the floors were outside their territory unless lights were there to attract the insects. This kind of lizard liked table salt, so they were given a Chinese name that meant "salt snake." In China, their mysterious name was "wall tiger."

Wall tigers have long served a medicinal purpose in China. After they are butchered and cleaned, they are dried over charcoal and then pulverized. This is later combined with other powdered substances such as musk, mercuric oxide, cinnabar, pearl, pinellia *(ban xia)*, and bezoar *(niu huang)*. The resultant powdered medicine is dissolved in water and administered orally. This is a popular and effective medicine for childhood cough and phlegm. Adults can take a cough remedy that is made by brewing wall tigers in wine for a month or so.

Bats lived under the eaves of every home in Cholon. At night, they came out in droves to chase after the insects. After several hours of feasting, they came back and rested in their sanctuaries. Bat excretion has long been used in Chinese medicine. After cleaning and then drying under the sun, bat excretion is called "night bright sand." This powdered medicine is widely used to cure weak night vision or night blindness. Older people with cataracts may avoid surgery by taking this medicine regularly. Night bright sand is generally included in a prescription with other herbs.

Geckos lived in the open spaces surrounding the homes. They ranged between half a foot to one foot, and resembled dark green lizards with dots. Their color would sometimes change into grey and purple. After butchering and removing their tails, the geckos are cleaned, dried, and then pulverized. The medicine is used to treat lung ailments such as tuberculosis. It is also effective for conditions due to old age such as weak knees, coughing, feeling constantly chilly despite adequate clothing, and frequent urination especially during the night. Gecko is usually a part of a prescription consisting of ginseng *(ren shen)*, glehnia *(sha shen)*, black dates, and honey.

The human residents of Cholon did not seem to be bothered by these three creatures. Their sanctuaries were never disrupted or destroyed. They were accepted as members of the ecosystem because they played a part in controlling the insect population.

Leprosy and Typhoid: Successful Treatment Approach Of The West

The chronic disease of leprosy occurs mostly in tropical and subtropical countries. When I was in Vietnam, the disease was believed to be contagious through physical contact. As a consequence, lepers were feared and isolated by the rest of the community. In Cholon, lepers would live together and care for one another in an isolated section of town rather than facing social rejection elsewhere.

There was no known cure for leprosy in Chinese medicine. I attempted to treat a few early-stage cases with herbs formulated to nourish the skin and the blood. However, the herbs could only provide temporary relief and were unable to control the disease. Leprosy first appears as reddish lesions under the skin, which gradually spread all over the body. The lesions cause a loss of sensation and slow degeneration of the tissues especially of the face, hands and feet. Left untreated, extreme disfigurement would result with the disappearance of the nose, ears, fingers, and toes.

The Saigon government attempted to contain and treat the disease in special hospitals, but with little result. American economic assistance to Vietnam in the 1960s funneled more resources to this project. The next few years saw a significant reduction of the leper population. Later I learned that Western medicine had discovered a cure for this disease, which is caused by the bacteria, *Mycobacterium leprae*. Thus, sulfonamides were introduced as a treatment for leprosy. Therapy was a long-term project involving education, isolation of the disease, chemotherapy, physiotherapy, and rehabilitation of patients after the disease was successfully controlled.

Unlike leprosy which slowly erodes the body without causing death directly, typhoid fever is a dangerous disease that can kill within a few months. Typhoid is common in developing countries due to poor sanitation. The disease is mainly transmitted through contaminated food or water. Symptoms at onset are a fever that appears to be ordinary, with associated fatigue, diarrhea, headache, cough, and loss of appetite. An ordinary fever goes away a few days after treatment. With typhoid, the fever persists and steadily worsens for another two weeks. The appearance of small red spots on the body is indicative of typhoid infection. If the patient receives timely treatment, the fever will gradually fade in two weeks. With severe cases, the high fever can last for two to three months, leading to perforation of the intestinal wall, heart failure, pneumonia, and acute inflammation of the gallbladder.

I remember one particular case of typhoid fever in which a man came to my home one evening. "I'd like you to come and treat my dying brother. He has been sick for three months." We sped off in a taxi to his home in Saigon. On the way, I gathered as much information as I could about the sick man's condition. Apparently, he had been treated by another herbalist but with no results. When we got there, the funeral company had already completed initial preparations. The patient had been dressed in funeral clothes and was laid in the middle of the living room for the moment of death to arrive.

When I touched Mr. Choi's forehead, hands, and abdomen, his high body temperature indicated the severity of the illness. He was very weak but conscious. Although he appeared to be dying, his pulse still exhibited some vitality. His tongue, despite a thick and yellow fur, did not show signs of major problems of the intestines or other vital organs. A person dying of typhoid would usually have a tongue that had turned dark. This was a severe case but the patient still had hope for recovery.

I asked the family to dress him back in regular clothes. There was some reluctance because the older family members were not convinced that the man would recover. I therefore proceeded to undress him while rebuking those present for failing to see the remaining vital signs of the patient. The patient's wife and his brother then assisted me in carrying him back to his room. We immediately used ice to cool his temperature.

For typhoid patients, the digestive system has difficulty absorbing food containing meat or oil. The best diet consists of frequent feeding of small quantities of thin rice soup with some sugar added. At the same time, the patient should be administered a prescription to cool the fever and cleanse the blood, with herbs such as forsythia *(lian qiao)*, phragmites *(lu gen)*, lophatherum *(zhu ye)*, and lysimachia *(jin qian cao)*. After such treatment, Mr. Choi gradually recovered within several weeks. His wife later thanked me for acting forcefully on that potentially fateful day.

A decade later, the incidence of typhoid was very much reduced, thanks to Western medicine. An antibiotic was developed to combat the bacteria, *Salmonella typhi,* which causes typhoid fever, and later, a vaccine was discovered.

Thus, Western medicine had invented a new method of treatment by directly attacking the agent of disease. Even though Chinese herbs are aimed at boosting the body's own defenses against the disease, they have shortcomings, especally in treating severe cases. With leprosy and typhoid fever, it was clear that Western medicine was far more effective in bringing about a rapid cure.

The Simple Good Life in Cholon

Due to geographic and cultural proximity, there long existed a special kinship between the peoples of China and Vietnam. Many older Vietnamese could speak and write Chinese. A large portion of the Vietnamese vocabulary was borrowed from Chinese although its alphabet was adopted from French. The Vietnamese government and the native people demonstrated generous accommodation and tolerance toward the large population of Chinese settlers. Cholon, which meant "big city," was probably the largest and most vibrant Chinatown that existed in any country outside of China.

The climate in Cholon was hot and humid all year round. In the early afternoon, the sun's heat forced most people to rest in the shade or take an afternoon nap. Consequently, the lunch hour was usually two hours or more. When the heat rose to an unbearable level, the rain would come to provide relief. During the monsoon season, heavy downpours lasted for a few hours, flooding the streets. When the rain clouds departed, the weather would turn cool for a day or so. In the night time after the rain dispelled the heat, everything seemed to come alive as one heard the humming and singing of all kinds of insects and other creatures. It reminded me of the pleasant life on a farm.

Food

Cholon offered a bounty of culinary enjoyment at low prices. Despite the on-going war in the countryside, food shortages occurred very seldom. In the morning, we never had to prepare breakfast at home. The food market on the next block offered a great variety of delicacies, both Chinese and Vietnamese. The question was not what was there to eat for breakfast, but what to choose. Our choices were from among a dozen kinds of noodles, rice porridge with different kinds of fresh seafood or meat, and some sweet delights to conclude the breakfast. At lunch and dinner, the market offered foods appropriate for those times. Then at night, fruits and light delicacies dominated as everyone went for a snack before going to bed. The food market stayed open until past midnight.

Sometimes, for a change, we would have a Western-style breakfast at a French bakery just around the corner. Or, when we were too lazy to walk the short distance to the food market, we would just sit at home and wait for the constant stream of food peddlers each of whom had a unique call to distinguish his or her specialty. During hot dry evenings, people on our street liked to relax outdoors in their rattan or wooden chairs in order to catch some cool breezes. I remember there was a woman peddler who sold *nem nuong*. She always found someone who wanted to place an order. She then sat next to the customer, started a small charcoal fire, and began barbecuing her marinated pork meat balls. The entire street was filled with the tempting smell of barbecued meat. Other neighbors quickly placed their orders. After a while, other food peddlers selling steamed sugar canes, fruits, and sweet delicacies converged. Before we realized it, we had a food festival on our street! This lasted for the entire evening before things finally returned normal.

Food peddlers were common in Cholon as well as in other developing countries. There was always concern about the cleanliness of the food. I always advised people to stay away from cold food and fruits that were already cut open, which could easily cause dysentery. However, cooked food was considered quite safe.

While the growing number of peddlers constituted the lower end of the retail food industry, the restaurant business in Vietnam also expanded rapidly. Most of the fancy French restaurants were located in Saigon less than forty-five minutes away by car. The one we liked to patronize was a floating restaurant on the Mekong River. Cafes were also common. Along the tree-lined streets in front of the Congress Building, it was pure delight to spend a lazy afternoon in a French-style sidewalk cafe watching the colorful traffic pass by on foot, bicycle, and motorcycle.

For Chinese food, Cholon boasted many fine restaurants, most of which served Cantonese cuisine. Larger restaurants could cater at customers' homes in the same tradition as in Canton. The restaurant would supply the personnel and equipment, and there was a choice between ready-made and made-in-the-home food. My mother-in-law who lived next door, liked to host birthday parties at home, and generally had the restaurant prepare the food at her house.

On the day of the party, the chefs, waitresses and assistants arrived in the early afternoon. They brought all the necessary equipment including caldrons, utensils, tables and chairs. It was fascinating to watch them set up a makeshift kitchen in the backyard. The best part came when they started to prepare the various dishes, including roasting a small pig, and the delicate preparation of a special soup to be steam-cooked inside a winter melon.

The guests began arriving in the late afternoon. The waitresses served them drinks and freshly-prepared cakes and appetizers. Usually the parties lasted until midnight. The restaurant personnel did the cleanup before they left. A dinner party at home cost not much more than at the restaurant mainly because of cheap labor. Best of all, it created a warm homey atmosphere.

Films, Cinemas, and Nightlife

Cholon did not have large museums or concert halls, but its cultural life was rich with its own simple traditions. Within a radius of one mile from our residence, we could count more than twenty movie theatres. They put on continuous shows between noon and 7 P.M.; an admission ticket entitled the viewer to stay for the entire time. During Sundays and holidays, the show started at 9 A.M. Theatres that had air-conditioning were filled with people seeking refuge from the hot afternoons.

There were basically four types of cinematic entertainment. The first kind, Cantonese movies and operas, were very popular with women and the older generation. The films were all imported from Hong Kong which, it is said, probably makes more movies than Hollywood. Most Cantonese productions were tragic love stories or folk tales that depicted the suffering of ordinary people caused by China's feudal society. These struck a chord with the audience, many of whom had probably been victims of the feudal system. My mother-in-law and her friends went to at least a couple of Cantonese movies every week. When they returned home, their eyes were red from crying. My wife liked those movies, too, but I managed to persuade her not to go so often, lest she became melancholy.

The second type, Mandarin movies, attracted the majority of the Chinese community, especially the young. These films were also imported from Hong Kong, and featured many entertainment talents from Shanghai. The period between 1955 and 1965 was considered the golden era of Mandarin movies. I can still remember the names of the movie kings and queens of that time. Unfortunately, most of them retired, passed away, or committed suicide at the zenith of their careers. Mandarin films were also shown in some theatres in Saigon where they attracted large Vietnamese audiences.

The third type of film were American ones, and were appreciated by both Vietnamese and Chinese audiences. Westerns and Disney animated movies were favorites in our family. Although films from France were also popular because of the French influence, American films were gradually eclipsing the French ones. The increasing popularity of the English language in Saigon also facilitated the acceptance of English movies.

Finally, there was an assortment of films imported from Japan and the Philippines, most of which were translated into Cantonese. The former were action-oriented centered around gang warfare and heroism. In the late 1950s, the story of an invisible man single-handedly battling the gangs was first featured in a Japanese movie. Films from the Philippines were rich in imagination and plot. One popular story was based on the theme of a superman.

Saigon's nightlife featured a variety of night clubs and bars in addition to the movie theatres. My wife and I sometimes left the children at home and went with friends to the night clubs in Saigon. We were all enthusiastic dancers. We waltzed, tangoed, and cha-cha'ed through the night before returning home in the early morning hours. The world seemed to be a happier place during the late 1950s and early 1960s. The entertainment field was going through a renaissance. To keep up with fashion, we had to learn a new dance every month, such as the mambo, rock and roll, and the stomach-wrenching twist.

The Growing American Influence

In the 1960s, the Beatlemania that swept America was carried over to Saigon by the American Armed Forces Radio. Within a couple of years, the establishment of a TV station by the Americans brought the visual images that profoundly transformed the thinking of the local residents. Because of an increasing American presence, the youths in Saigon caught on to whatever was hot in America within weeks. The emergence of rock and roll, rhythm and blues, surfing music, and folk songs, and their accompanying craze reflected the simple and happy life of that period.

In America, disillusion with the Vietnam war gave rise to anti-war sentiment. The hippie movement and the use of drugs as an escape were expressions of disenchanted youths. I could understand the feeling of powerlessness among the young. The older generation occupied all the seats of power, and made a grave mistake by sending the young generation to a questionable war of attrition in a faraway land. What could the young people do except protest and rebel in their own way? Although I sympathized with the young, I did not condone using drugs as an escape. The hippie movement did not find a following in Saigon except for the long-hair look.

Besides pop music, American culture was imparted to Vietnam through the import of automobiles. Cars made in Detroit added a great deal of color to the streets of Saigon and Cholon. They dwarfed the smaller Renaults and Citroens made in France. The modern design of a Cadillac convertible and other American

makes often attracted a crowd of curious and admiring onlook-
ers. The wealthy were switching to the conspicuous and trendy
American models. Some of my friends owned an American car. I
was impressed by the styling, the smooth ride, and the automat-
ic transmission which was a new invention then. With the added
reputation of high fuel consumption, the American automobile
immediately translated into wealth, fashion, and prestige for the
local people.

My wife and children had desired a private car for some time.
One evening, a salesman whom I knew drove over a huge Buick
with large high tail fins to take us for a ride. The children were
filled with excitement as they jumped into the car. It was a fine
ride, but I had my own reservations. I had never wanted to drive
a car, for the disorderly traffic frightened me. My diminutive wife
probably could not even see over the hood of that big vehicle, let
alone learn how to drive it. On our way back after stopping off at
the car dealer to pick up some more information, I cautioned the
children to keep their hands away from the door before I closed
It. "Ouch!" I caught my own hand instead. The salesman was
embarrassed by the accident and quickly drove us home. Three
fingers of mine turned swollen and black, but luckily no bones
were broken. This incident gave me a good excuse to postpone
the car issue. The rest of the family did not bring it up again.

Home Entertainment and the Japanese Influence

The activity I enjoyed most was to throw a music party at home.
Once or twice a month, I invited a dozen friends over for the
evening. They brought along their string and pipe instruments,
and I sang to their accompaniment well into the night. The neighbors did not mind, and ended up coming over for a free concert
of Cantonese opera. At 10 P.M., we had an intermission and served
snacks which usually included sweet soup, a popular sweet broth

made from a variety of foods. The Cantonese believed in the nourishing effect of sweet soup, especially for the lungs, the throat, and
the skin.

To play music at a party was fun; to record and play it back
later provided a higher level of enjoyment. I owned a tape recorder
made by the famous Grundig Company of Germany. One day,
the shop owner who sold me this recorder asked me to go over to
see his new products. The new sound technology called stereo was
being incorporated into the tape recorder for the first time. The
latest Grundig model was twice as big as mine, and had four speak-
ers and two microphones. After listening to it, I thought it was an
impressive piece of technology.

Then the shop owner led me to a separate room to see the "real
thing." It looked like a black robot sitting upright on the table. I
saw the name Akai and asked if it was made in America. "This is
made in Japan. What do you think?" I had never been impressed
by the Japanese before except for their firepower and ferocity. We
sat down and listened to the beautiful sound which far surpassed
that of the Grundig at the same price. It suddenly dawned on me
that a second Japanese invasion had already begun. This one was
economic as opposed to the military one some twenty years ago.
I needed no more sales pitch to settle for the Akai. After I brought
it home, the living room was turned into a display hall as the neighbors came to marvel at the "little monster."

Within a few years, Japanese products were everywhere. In the
home, Japan had a monopoly on rice cookers and dominated the
market in electric fans. We had replaced the German Grundig
recorder with the Akai, the Dutch Philips radio with a Sony, and
the American RCA record player with a National. Our second
refrigerator was a Sanyo replacing a European make. We did not
see any Japanese cars in the streets, yet. As for motorcycles, the
French Solex and the Italian Vespa were giving way to the Honda,
the Suzuki, and the Yamaha. Soon, television sets, air condition-
ers, and washing machines were added to the long list of Japanese

products. The Japanese had successfully ousted other competitors from Vietnam and other Southeast Asian countries, which had constituted Japan's first export markets and provided them with valuable international marketing experience. Who could have imagined at that time that Japanese automobiles would capture close to 25 percent of the American market twenty more years later?

Festivals and Celebrations

Like Canton, Cholon was rich in Chinese tradition. The most important festival was, of course, the Chinese Lunar New Year, which the Vietnamese celebrated as Tet. Almost all businesses were closed for a whole week. Fewer people seemed to get sick then and the number of my patients dwindled considerably. Children especially loved this festival because parents traditionally relaxed the household rules. There were only a few things to do: eat, play, go to the movies, and visit friends round the clock. Preparation for the New Year ordinarily took three weeks; recovering from it took another week. Then came the Dragon Boat Festival in May, the Ghost Festival in July, followed by the Mid-Autumn Festival. In between these major celebrations, there were Christmas and countless Buddhist festivals, enough to allow work breaks and renewal of the body and soul.

Even the natural death of a person was cause for celebration. My mother joined me in Cholon around 1954. She passed away in 1961 at the age of eighty. The funeral company provided a package of services including three days of homage and celebration at home, a group of Buddhist priests to conduct prayers, a funeral procession with a band, and finally, burial in the cemetery. A temporary structure was erected in front of our house which required pedestrians to detour. The body was clothed in funereal dress and placed in a wooden coffin in the middle of the living room. All the relatives and friends came to pay their respects. The monks chanted their prayers at regular intervals. The ceremony lasted round the clock for three days. Close relatives and friends stayed overnight and helped with the organization of activities. This was the best occasion when one could meet and entertain all the friends at home within a short period of time.

Excursions Outside the City

Although the Saigon-Cholon area had much to offer, we regularly ventured to other cities by car. Our most frequent destination was Thu Duc, a pleasant half-day holiday for our family and the herb store employees. We usually chartered a taxi, and drove along a highway that cut through huge rubber plantations. We arrived in a Vietnamese restaurant that was essentially a villa with a large swimming pool that drew its water from nearby creeks and wells. There, we just ate, swam, napped, or hiked along the trails.

One of Vietnam's best vacation resorts was Dalat in the Central Highlands. The journey took about nine hours by car, but the overnight train was the most relaxing mode of transport. It left Saigon station in the afternoon and wound through the wild countryside. In some locations, we were warned to keep the windows shut and not to wander outside the carriage when the train stopped, for fear of tigers waiting in the bushes and preying on the straying passengers. At one point, the train stopped for the passengers to view the ancient mountain tribes whose scantily clad members still engaged in hunting with spears and arrows. In the morning, the train began a steep climb. The scenery was both terrific and terrifying. The slow-moving train seemed to be hanging on the side of the cliff. Looking out, we only saw rocks, trees and waterfalls hundreds of feet below.

Due to the high altitude, Dalat's climate was autumn-like year round. The tourist focal point was a beautiful lake in the city. The French had built elegant bungalows along the shore. We loved to circumnavigate the lake in a rented horse-carriage, and to paddle-boat on the calm waters. Another outdoor activity in Dalat was deer hunting. Some restaurants specialized in deer meat, and allowed customers into their slaughter houses to pick the fresh catch of the day. Some of Vietnam's largest waterfalls were located in Dalat.

As the war heated up, travel through the countryside became increasingly dangerous. We did not venture out of town anymore after 1965. We heard many horror stories about motorists being caught in cross fire. One of the worst things that could happen was if Vietcong were found to be near a highway, a light spotter plane would mark the location with smoke in the sky. A few minutes later, American jets from nearby bases would drop napalm bombs on the area.

How The War Evolved

Japan took over Vietnam from France between 1942 and 1945. When Japan surrendered, the Vietnamese nationalists led by Ho Chi Minh proclaimed the country's independence. The Vietnamese nationalist movement had been nurtured and supported by the Chinese Communist Party which was then fighting a long civil war in mainland China. France was opposed to Vietnamese independence and sent troops to regain control of her former colony. In 1949, France reinstated the Vietnamese emperor, Bao Dai, but retained actual governing power. Ho led a protracted guerrilla war which culminated in the French defeat at Dien Bien Phu in 1954. The United Nations intervened and divided Vietnam along the 17th parallel to enforce a cease-fire: the north to be ruled by Ho Chi Minh and the south by Bao Dai. France then began her final disengagement from Vietnam.

In 1955, Prime Minister Ngo Dinh Diem engineered a referendum that abolished the monarchy of Bao Dai. Ngo became the first president of the Republic of South Vietnam. In 1956, Ngo refused to participate in the general election throughout Vietnam as agreed to by both sides earlier in the Geneva Accords to determine if the country could be unified under one government. With the election cancelled, the Communists from the north began infiltrating the south in support of the local Vietcong to seek unification by force.

Fearing the spread of communism in Asia, the United States readily came to South Vietnam's assistance. By the end of 1961, U.S. military advisors had increased from several hundred to 18,000 who took on fighting responsibility if necessary. Ngo's authoritarian government failed to make significant progress on both the economic and military fronts. Furthermore, he antagonized the popular Buddhist church. The monks protested by setting themselves on fire one after another in the streets of Saigon, an event that captured world headlines. It was widely rumored that President Kennedy ordered the CIA to plot Ngo's removal. In early November 1963, Ngo was killed in a military coup. The U.S. involvement in Vietnam deepened. Vietcong insurgency increased correspondingly. The instability of the Saigon government was marked by frequent reshuffling at the highest level.

The war in Vietnam escalated. By 1969, U.S. troops there numbered over half a million. The United States managed to gain some international support. South Korea committed around 47,000 troops; Australia and New Zealand to a much less extent. In addition, the U.S. navy carried out daily bombing missions against North Vietnam from its aircraft carriers offshore. The U.S. air force employed giant B-52 bombers based in Guam, the Philippines, and Thailand for frequent carpet bombings of communist concentrations and supply routes. The prospect was real that North Vietnam could be reduced to the stone age as threatened by U.S. General LeMay.

There was little doubt that the United States could win the war with her overwhelming might. However, the world would soon be reminded that a war was planned by people, fought by people, and won by people. Technology and weaponry were only one of many factors that bring victory under certain circumstances.

The Communists were growing stronger day by day. The usual guerrilla warfare sometimes erupted into battles supported by tanks on both sides below the 17th parallel. In the south, the Vietcong controlled the countryside. The Saigon government controlled the major cities. The Americans controlled the military bases along the coast and adjacent to the major cities. The cities and the bases were in fact isolated islands in a sea of enemy territory.

The War Hits Home

It was clear that the war was approaching closer to home. After midnight, we frequently heard the thunder of sustained bombings in the outskirts of Cholon. Sometimes, the horizon would light up and we would feel the concussion shortly afterward. Later, we learned that those were B-52 bombing raids from an altitude of over 30,000 feet. The bombers could neither be seen nor heard, but they brought enormous destruction to the target area. There were usually no reports about the number of enemy killed, nor about the civilian casualties. We only learned from the news that Vietcong concentrations had been neutralized to allow U.S. and South Vietnamese troops to continue their search-and-destroy missions.

As more American servicemen arrived, more accommodations were needed in Saigon. Hotels were rented or purchased for conversion to military quarters. A few blocks from our residence in Cholon, one hotel was converted for American servicemen, and another for their Australian counterparts. The concentration of foreign military personnel was an invitation to Vietcong terrorist attacks with grenades or plastic bombs. This led to the Americans sealing off the areas surrounding the hotel buildings and the positioning of armed guards at strategic locations. The fortressed hotels created a high level of tension in the neighborhood. As residents, we could only circumvent that forbidden area for safety's sake. In my mind, I worried about the prospects of this war. After all these years, it had evolved from guerrilla warfare restricted to the countryside to almost an urban conflict. Now we did not feel safe even in the capital.

The Tet Offensive Shakes My Faith

In late January 1968, the Communists launched the Tet (lunar new year) offensive against all the major cities of South Vietnam. Even the heavily-defended U.S. embassy in Saigon was attacked. The fighting in Cholon was fierce. We fled to safety in another district of town when we saw South Vietnamese troops with artillery and tanks moving into the neighborhood, supported by U.S. helicopter gunships hovering above. We also had a first glimpse of the fighting men and women of the Vietcong as they came out of nowhere and assembled for the house-to-house fighting.

The street battle in Cholon lasted for several days. When we returned, a repulsive smell of dead bodies hung over the neighborhood. My herb shop was partially destroyed. Fei, an employee who lived there, was killed. Our house still stood but was ransacked. Most of the houses already had a bomb shelter built underneath a couple of years ago. My mother-in-law was lost in the confusion of the evacuation. She and another relative had lived through the street battle inside the shelter. We thought that she was probably dead. When I saw her emerging from the shelter, I ran toward her, embraced her, and cried.

The Tet offensive showed the world that the Vietcong could strike whenever and wherever they wanted. The only consolation was that the popular uprising expected by the Communists did not materialize. Washington finally came to realize that the war could not possibly be won, although the military commanders continued to request more troops. President Nixon, newly elected in late 1968 with a mandate to end the war, began the Vietnamization process which involved a phased withdrawal of all American land forces from South Vietnam. The horrors of the Tet

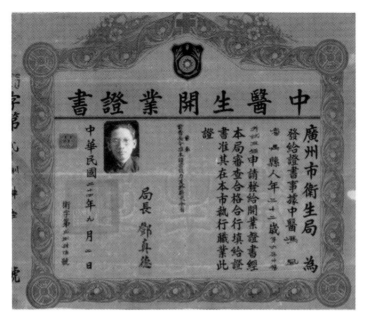

Dr. Fung's license in Canton.

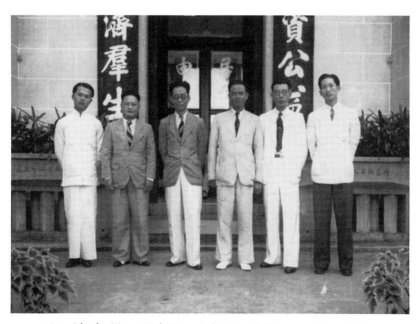

Outside the Tung Wah Hospital in South Vietnam circa 1940.
Dr. Fung is the first on the right.

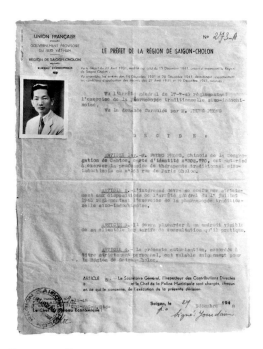

Dr. Fung's license in South Vietnam, 1948.

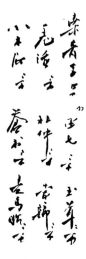

An arthritis formula from Dr. Fung's practice
(also reproduced on the cover).

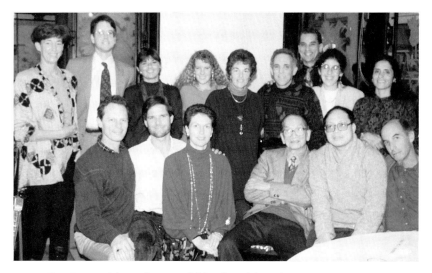

Dr. Fung with students and friends at his retirement party, 1993.

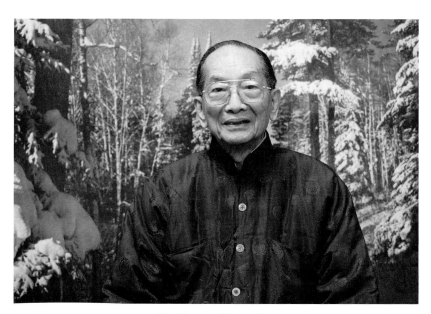

Dr. Fung at Yosemite.

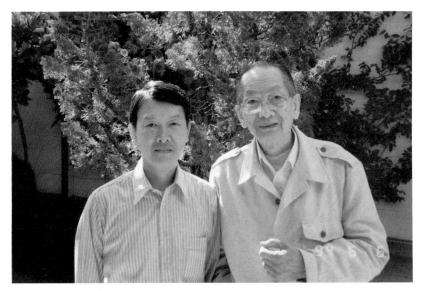

The two authors, John Fung and Dr. Fung.

offensive was only more of an encouragement to leave the country in spite of my business success. Our two sons had already left for Hong Kong several years ago. My wife, her mother, and our two daughters left for Hong Kong later in 1968. I was now committed to leaving as well.

America's heavy involvement in Vietnam greatly impacted the ordinary local residents. The most obvious influence was the establishment of the Armed Forces Radio which broadcast the latest news and American music. Many teenagers including my children developed a craze for American pop music. Later, the Americans ushered in television when they set up a station in Saigon. The first freeway was built between Saigon and Bien Hoa Air Base which became a showpiece of American technology and progress. Many youngsters began learning English rather than French as a second language, and they aspired to go to the United States for higher education. The French-made city buses were replaced by ones made in Detroit. Some streets were filled with bars and brothels catering to American servicemen. A black market of U.S. military supplies flourished in the streets of Saigon.

The American influence was not only materialistic. I recall one incident that occurred at a busy intersection when the traffic light broke down. The scene was a mess as the drivers honked and yelled at one another. A U.S. Army jeep pulled up. An American military policeman rushed to the intersection and began directing traffic. The drivers were pleased to see an authority trying to restore order. At the same time, there were two Vietnamese policemen standing on one corner of the intersection. They just watched and chatted away. To a significant extent, this interesting street scene explained why America lost the war. The intended joint effort between South Vietnam and the United States eventually deteriorated into American takeover of almost everything that the South Vietnamese government should have done for its own citizens.

As the war heated up, the Saigon government was drafting earnest young men for the army. I began to worry about my two sons' safety when they turned thirteen. Our neighbor's son had joined an elite group of the South Vietnamese army and was killed in action after just three months. We had heard stories about bicycle riders in the streets being rounded up by the police as a new conscription law went into effect. I wanted to send my sons to Hong Kong where my brother and sister were living. At that time, leaving South Vietnam required an exit visa from the Foreign Ministry. The chances of a teenager obtaining an exit visa were very small because of the draft requirement.

A native Vietnamese friend of mine told me that he had some connections with a high official in the Foreign Ministry who might be able to help get an exit visa for my eldest son who was approaching fifteen years of age. The friend arranged for a dinner meeting in a nice restaurant. The deal was sealed for the price of 30,000 Vietnamese piastres. Two years later, my second son obtained an exit visa for 50,000 piastres. Another friend of mine had to pay half a million for his nineteen-year-old son. By the late 1960s, there was an open market for exit visas. Some unlucky people paid the wrong officials who did not have the power to secure an exit visa. Many young men who could not afford payment escaped the draft by fleeing to Phnom Penh in neighboring Cambodia, where the Chinese embassy issued passports for them to go to China via Hong Kong. Many of them ended up staying in Hong Kong as illegal immigrants.

Departing With Sad Memories

In 1969, two days before my departure, my close friends invited me to a farewell dinner. The food looked delicious but everyone was in a somber mood. A waiter brought over a large bowl of shark-fin soup and prepared to set it in the center of the table. The bowl suddenly broke. Everyone was caught by surprise. The owner of the restaurant immediately came and apologized. The breaking of glass on such an occasion was a bad omen in Chinese tradition, as it implied the destruction of something dear to everyone present such as closeness and partnership. All of us tried to ignore what had happened. For most of us, it was the last supper we had together.

On the day I left, my mind was filled with sad reflections. As I rode to the airport, I saw groups of young American servicemen gathering in their favorite spots in the streets of Saigon. They had been sent to a faraway land to safeguard democracy and protect the security of the United States. The noble meaning of democracy was hardly tenable in the case of South Vietnam. The national security of the United States was ill-defined by Washington. American intervention was based on the unfounded fear of the spread of communism in Asia.

After involvement, U.S. intelligence overestimated their own firepower, but neglected the will and tenacity of the enemy. They also overestimated the capability of the South Vietnamese government in delivering reforms. By the end of the war, more than 50,000 Americans would never return home. Others would suffer for the rest of their lives the injuries and trauma incurred during the war. As a parent who hated to see children die for a dubious cause, my heart impulsively went out to those whom I did not know but had lost their loved ones in this tragic war.

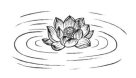

Chapter 5

Hong Kong 1969–1979: Temporary Shelter Again

A Successful Colony

Hong Kong had changed beyond recognition upon my return after thirty years. One could easily feel the heartbeat of capitalism thriving in this British colony of about six million people. The success of Hong Kong is the result of a unique interplay of political and economic forces shaping East and Southeast Asia.

When Japanese troops left in August 1945, Britain reclaimed its former colony of Hong Kong, ignoring the protest from the Nationalist government struggling for survival on the Chinese mainland. The British re-occupation was made easy thanks to the non-existence of an independence movement in Hong Kong. In October 1949 when the Communists won the final victory over the Nationalists on the Chinese mainland, Britain was among the first to extend recognition to the People's Republic of China. The Communist troops advanced to Canton but stopped at the border with Hong Kong, thus guaranteeing the status quo of the Colony for the next few decades.

During the 1950s, the world saw a wave of de-colonization and the emergence of a growing number of independent states. China delivered a message to the United Nations emphasizing the special political status of Hong Kong and opposing any international attempt to foster its independence. This position has never been challenged by the world community. China had maintained that the political status of Hong Kong would be settled when the time was ripe. That time finally came in 1984 when Britain and China signed an agreement for the return of the Colony to Chinese rule in July 1997. The agreement for two governments to change hands peacefully with neither significant support nor opposition from the local residents was indeed a rare phenomenon in modern history.

The people of Hong Kong may exhibit little interest in politics and government, but they embrace capitalism with utmost enthusiasm. The economy of Hong Kong was originally founded on entrepot trade between China and the rest of the world. At the close of the civil war in China when the Communists appeared to be winning, many industrialists left Shanghai and settled in Hong Kong, thus laying the foundation for a manufacturing industry. This manufacturing base later developed into a world-class consumer industry, exporting products such as clothing, toys and electronics mostly to the developed countries of North America and Western Europe.

In the latter half of the 1980s just when the principal export markets of Hong Kong were heading toward a recession, the Nationalist government in Taiwan relaxed travel and investment restrictions with regard to China. Due to the absence of a direct transportation link, millions of Taiwan residents had to pass through Hong Kong on their way to and from the Mainland. This has greatly benefited Hong Kong, especially the tourist and related industries. The overtures between the two Chinese governments on opposite sides of the Taiwan Strait without formal recognition has produced a windfall for the Hong Kong economy. This situation will probably last for some time as the two sides engage in on-and-off negotiations trying to establish some sort of direct communication link.

The single most important development since the late 1980s is China's opening of its coastal regions to foreign investment. This presents a golden opportunity for Hong Kong to solve once and for all its chronic problems of labor shortage, high land and raw material costs. As a consequence, Hong Kong capital flows into China like water through an open dam. Many factories have relocated or expanded their production to Shenzhen and other cities across the border. In addition, Chinese investment in the Colony has also increased significantly due to economic liberalization on the Mainland. Even before its official reversion to Chinese rule, Hong Kong has in fact largely integrated its economy with that of the Greater Canton Region.

Economic integration with southern China is the best long-term insurance policy for Hong Kong's stability and survival. Because of its dynamic economic development, southern China, especially Guangdong province, will amass more clout and bargaining power as time elapses. Southern China has already gained exemptions and favorable treatment from the central government in Beijing. The identification and integration of Hong Kong with southern China will only secure its future.

The other insurance policy that Hong Kong has is China's pursuit of peaceful reunification with Taiwan. Because Taiwan has a strong defense force equipped with modern American weapons, reunification by force would prove costly. On the other hand, reunification talks attempted previously have resulted in deadlock and frustration. China's proposal of a "one country two systems" formula has always been viewed by Taiwan with great suspicion. Should the situation in Hong Kong remain stable and prosperous after 1997, Taiwan would be more inclined to pursue the reunification talks. Therefore, if peaceful reunification remains a top priority as it is now, China will have every reason to maintain the thriving capitalist system in Hong Kong as a model to placate Taiwan.

However, a major uncertainty that has recently surfaced is the democratization of Taiwan's political system. In the new Legislative Assembly, the Democratic Progressive Party (DPP) has captured almost one-third of the seats versus a slight majority won by the ruling Nationalist Party. The DPP has grass-root support from the island natives and is a champion of Taiwan independence. China has repeatedly threatened to use force should Taiwan declare itself an independent state. If the political development in Taiwan continues its present course favoring the DPP, it is possible that a major war could erupt in the Taiwan Strait, an event that would destabilize all of East Asia.

The stable and open banking industry in Hong Kong has attracted huge amounts of capital from Chinese settlers in Southeast Asia. Between 1950 and 1980, Southeast Asian countries were plagued by various types of instability. The notable ones were communist insurgency in Malaysia, Vietnam, Cambodia, Thailand, and Laos; bloody racial riots in Malaysia; and the large-scale purges of Chinese communities in Indonesia after a failed communist coup attempt in 1965. Thus, wealthy Chinese settlers considered Hong Kong a Switzerland of the East where they could safely deposit their money.

I myself began to funnel my savings into Hong Kong in the early 1960s when the Vietnam war started to escalate. At that time, foreign exchange restrictions were already in place which limited remittances to very small amounts. The official exchange rate was one Hong Kong dollar to about fifteen Vietnamese piastres. However, there were other remittance channels available at twice the official exchange rate. This was still reasonable considering the absence of other alternatives and the depreciating piastre.

A travel agent I knew had connections with some export-import houses in both Hong Kong and Cholon. I delivered the piastres to this travel agent in Cholon. Two weeks later, an import house in Hong Kong called my sister to pick up the Hong Kong dollars I wanted to remit. The travel agent told me that he used the piastres to buy Vietnamese raw materials, then sold them to the Hong Kong importer, who also got a list of the payees for payment in Hong Kong dollars. All transactions on the Vietnamese side were done in cash. I can still remember my petite wife carrying three bags of cash and riding off to the travel agent in a taxi. The driver offered to help load the "baggage" but my wife nervously refused. The remittances were solely based on trust with no receipts for proof. All transactions were executed smoothly and confidentially.

The outflow of money from Vietnam to Hong Kong was due to a war. There was also an outflow of money from Hong Kong to other countries, particularly Canada and the United States. The political uncertainty in Hong Kong was the major reason. The open banking and financial system in Hong Kong placed no restrictions on the amount of remittances, hence only one official exchange rate applied. Since the early 1960s when the Cultural Revolution began in China, many Hong Kong residents started opening foreign accounts overseas as a hedge.

Foreign consulates in Hong Kong also received increasing numbers of applications for immigrant visas. In 1982 after China officially demanded negotiation for the return of Hong Hong to Chinese sovereignty, the lines for immigrant visas spilled into the streets at the American and some other consulates. Canada has been most successful in attracting Hong Kong manpower and capital as evidenced by the real estate developments in Vancouver and Toronto. Australia has lately become a popular destination. Now, in the 1990s, many Hong Kong professionals hold Canadian or Australian passports. Despite the outflow of talent and capital, the economy of Hong Kong continues to flourish due to its integration with the booming Chinese economy.

Resuming Practice in Hong Kong

After settling in Hong Kong, I was introduced by a friend to the owner of an herb store in Mong Kok District. Mr. Chao asked if I wanted to join him as a resident physician in his store. Our partnership was to last for the next ten years.

Fibroids: There Is An Alternative To Surgery

Surgery is an expensive procedure in Western medicine. Many Chinese are fearful of surgery. The traditional thinking is that surgery, although successful, will do irreparable damage to the Source Qi of the body, just like an opened can of soft drink will lose some of its carbonation. Source Qi is considered the innate collective vital energy of the body. A gradual and irreversible dissipation of Source Qi takes place over a lifetime until its full depletion at death. Surgery opens up a part of the body and accelerates this dissipation of vital energy.

The above traditional thinking may be mystifying, but the stress of going through surgery is real. Surgery requires extensive tests and preparation. Anesthetics and other drugs that are administered produce varying degrees of side effects. Recovery may extend over a long time during which the patient must gradually learn to adjust. Therefore, the benefits of surgery should be weighed against all the costs. In contrast, Chinese medicine offers cures for non-acute conditions at a low cost and devoid of unpleasant side effects.

At a wedding banquet of a friend in 1970, an elderly woman came to me and asked if I remembered her. In an effort to refresh my memory, I inquired about her name and family profession. However, I still could not recall who she was. "I was one of your patients some forty years ago!" That really gave me a pleasant surprise. Mrs. Chai then recounted that she had had a uterine fibroid around 1939 when I was practising in Hong Kong. A Western doctor had recommended surgery but she was frightened by the idea. She consulted me for a prescription and took the herbs regularly for almost one year. The fibroid gradually disappeared.

Fibroids are not uncommon. They are benign tumors occurring on or in the uterine wall, and usually affect women between thirty and fifty years of age. From a Chinese medical point of view, fibroids are caused by a deficiency of Yang in the blood. Thus, taking herbs that nourish the blood and tonify the Yang will gradually eliminate the tumors.

Menstrual Conditions

Menstrual conditions occur in women at different ages. One day a Miss Liang was carried on the back of her mother to the herb shop. The young lady was sixteen years old. She was crying because of the great pain in her abdomen. I touched it and it felt hard, suggesting muscle tension. She indicated more pain when I applied force. There were no signs that the pain originated from any of the vital organs. I read her pulse, it was quick and strong, which was typical of people with high blood pressure. The pulse also indicated the existence of excess Heat inside the body. She did not have a fever but felt very warm in the abdomen. There were also no signs of organ malfunction.

I diagnosed the condition as a menstrual problem. I asked if she had menstruated yet. She answered never. I told her and her mother that she was about to have her first period. It was delayed because of the muscle tension in the uterus. The tension was the root cause of the pain. I wrote a prescription aimed at relaxing the muscles and promoting the menstrual flow. During the next few days, the girl in fact had her first period. The abdominal pain was alleviated as well.

Another case involved a Mrs. Chu who was in her thirties. She had had excessive menstruation for three days. The loss of blood rendered her pale, tired, and dizzy. Her pulse was relatively weak. In addition, she felt pain in the lower abdomen which was due to muscle tension. I used gelatin *(e jiao)*, myrrh *(mo yao)*, and frankincense *(ru xiang)* in my prescription to reduce the bleeding and relieve the pain. The prescription also contained other herbs that promoted her blood circulation, relaxed the muscles, and replenished the Qi.

Another common menstrual problem is experienced by women going through menopause, which is the cessation of menstruation that usually occurs after age forty-five. Menopausal women often experience physical and emotional stress. During the menopause which may last for many months, the physical stress can include irregular menstruation, loss of appetite, numbness of the limbs, nightsweats, insomnia, dizziness, a mild roaring sound in the ears, and sudden onset and dissipation of heat known as hot flashes. The emotional stress involves the anxiety associated with the menopause, which in the minds of many women, implies the onset of old age and the loss of productivity. Thus, depression and fluctuating emotions may set in. The physical discomforts of menopause can intensify the emotional stress and vice versa.

Menopause is not an illness but a natural physiologic process. Therefore, treatment should not interfere with this process. Instead, it should be aimed at resolving the physical and mental stress. Chinese treatment of menopause emphasizes easing this physical transition. A delicate balance of herbs that regulate the blood flow, restoring the functional balance of the organs, especially of the kidneys and the liver, will usually help alleviate the symptoms of menopause.

Diabetes: Inexpensive Supplemental Treatment

Diabetes is a chronic disease caused by a malfunction of the pancreas which results in deficiency of the hormone, insulin. The symptoms are frequent urination, thirst, weakness, itching, hunger, weight loss, and high sugar content in the blood.

I remember one such case, a Mr. Hui who was a government employee in his mid-thirties. He had been receiving Western treatment for his diabetes in a government clinic for three years. Besides adhering to a strict diet, he received regular urine testing and hormone injections to keep the disease in check. Unfortunately, the side effects of the medication had taken their toll. Mr. Hui was particularly distressed by the future possibility of going through the painful process of dialysis and of having to carry a dialysis machine wherever he went.

Mr. Hui came to me to explore an alternative. I explained to him that the approach of Chinese medicine was completely different. Instead of interventions such as injections or dialysis, Chinese herbs would act on the spleen and the kidneys to regulate the diuretic process of the body. The purpose was to assist the organs in performing their proper functions. I assured him that the herbs would produce few side effects. Furthermore, the traditional modality would not interfere with the Western treatment he was receiving.

Mr. Hui came to me regularly for one year or so, and took the herbal prescription three times a week. During this time, the diabetes remained under control, and the symptoms gradually improved. Mr. Hui was especially happy when the government clinic recommended that he probably would not need any dialysis. This was a case where Chinese and Western medicine could complement each other to alleviate the patient's suffering. Mr. Hui became a good friend of mine. Several years later, his diabetes had been reduced to a minor ailment, and through a careful diet and occasional treatment, it remained so.

Natural Beauty Is The Best

Miss Yu was an accountant in her mid-twenties, and led an active social life. Her lifestyle involved frequenting restaurants, night-clubs, and the movies. She was very conscious about how she dressed and the way she looked. Besides her social activities, her life was filled with irregular schedules. Occasional heavy work-loads required her to work well after midnight for a few days straight. When the work subsided, she was busy with the nightlife. As a consequence, she suffered from various minor ailments such as constipation, indigestion, irregular menstruation, and insomia. She appeared quite pale without her makeup. She lacked energy and was irritable. So she turned to various over-the-counter reme-dies to alleviate her ailments.

Miss Yu came to me on her friends' recommendations. She wanted some herbs that would improve her health and make her look more beautiful. Miss Yu needed a formula that would regu-late her body functions to bring about normal health. She took my prescription twice a week. After a month or so, she reported that she felt much better overall. Because her health improved, she had more confidence and enjoyed life more. Her paleness also dis-appeared gradually, and as a result, she did not have to put on so much makeup to mask it.

Another woman, Mrs. Chan, was a middle-aged housewife. Her routine housework gave her little time for recreation except for watching television. Sometimes she felt bored and low-spirit-ed. Her husband was a businessman who was on frequent assign-ments out of town. The little time they had together was not particularly filled with excitement. She thought that her husband had lost interest in her because she was aging. She pointed at some wrinkles on her face and the dryness of her skin, and wondered if Chinese herbs could help her skin look better.

The case of Mrs. Chan did not involve any illness. She just needed some herbs to consolidate the Yin in her body, energize the blood circulation, and nourish the skin. She took the pre-scription twice a week for many months, and reported that the herbs had restored her to normal appearance. Her skin gradually became moist and soft. She also mentioned that one time her hus-band asked why she suddenly appeared more attractive than before.

Beauty does not necessarily require cosmetics, nice clothes, or plastic surgery. A woman wants to have good health and be energetic and confident. This is what natural beauty is all about. Chinese herbs are able to enhance the beauty and femininity of a woman by improving her health and complexion. There is no doubt that the condition of a person's health determines the appearance, confidence, and behavior of that person.

Lack Of Energy

Mr. Cho was an office worker in his early thirties. He was pale, lacked appetite, and was underweight. His work seemed to be drowning him. He slept for over ten hours a day but still lacked energy. He showed little interest in other things besides work and television. After seeing me, Mr. Cho took my prescription daily. He felt better after a few days and wondered if he could continue with the herbs. I advised that since the herbs were natural, he could continue with the prescription, but that twice a week would suffice.

A few months later, Mr. Cho came by my office to say hello. He told me that he felt like a different person. In fact, he had clearly gained weight. He said that he was participating in many different activities including the YMCA sports program, and was an active member of a neighborhood church. I advised that by keeping up with his new activities, he would not need the prescription anymore.

Another one of my patients, Mr. Hu, was a recent retiree in his early sixties. He was unaccustomed to life that was without a regular schedule. He found himself staying at home and napping most of the time. The more he napped, the less interest he had for doing other things. He tried to read but could not concentrate for long. He could not amass the energy to even engage in gardening, his longtime hobby. Mr. Hu took my prescription for two weeks and the herbs gave him enough lift to adjust to his new lifestyle. He was able to divide his time between gardening, reading, and exercising.

Lack of energy or feeling apathetic is a common phenomenon when the Yin and Yang are not in tune. This means that the vital organs do not perform in harmony, and blood circulation is not at its best. Consequently, the Qi of the body is suppressed. Natural herbs will restore the organs and the body to normal performance.

The Agony Of Family Separation

In my generation, many Chinese families have to endure the agony of family separation due to war and economic depression. When I was young, my father had to leave Canton and work in Hong Kong out of economic necessity. I always treasured the times when he rejoined us in Canton during his brief leaves.

It is easy to take family togetherness for granted until a member has to leave for some reason. Just like good health, one seldom appreciates its value until one loses it. In 1962, our family faced the agony of separation when our eldest son of fifteen had to leave to avoid the possibility of being drafted into the South Vietnamese army. Two years later, our second son also left for Hong Kong. In 1968, my wife, her mother, and our two daughters left for Hong Kong. After closing my business in Cholon, I came to Hong Kong to join them in 1969. However, shortly before I arrived, my mother-in-law died of a heart attack. Then the two boys left us again to pursue their college educations in the United States. Thus, since 1962, our family has never had the chance of being together except for two brief periods in 1971 and 1975 when our sons came home to visit us.

My wife was especially saddened by this long period of family separation. Her total devotion to our children had taxed every bit of her energy. She worried constantly about the well-being of our children, especially our sons who had left her care when they were only teenagers. Many times I saw her weep after reading the weekly letters from the boys. I tried to comfort her by telling her that the boys knew how to take care of themselves. The worry and depression gradually weakened her health. She later developed anorexia and passed away in 1978. I had cured many people in my life, but to my deepest sorrow, I had failed to cure my most beloved one.

By 1978, my eldest son had been settled in San Francisco for many years. He wanted the entire family to join him. I had never imagined myself to be living in the United States before. Although I could speak and write some English, I knew it would be a cultural shock for me at the age of seventy. However, there was nothing more precious than being together with the family once again. In the spring of 1979, I left Hong Kong for the United States. I was probably one of the oldest immigrants to enter the country.

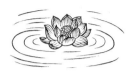

Chapter 6

San Francisco 1979–1994: My Permanent Home

The New Life In America

Americans enjoy one of the highest standards of living in the world. Although the quality of life can be viewed from many angles, Americans are blessed by the open spaces, a temperate climate, a generally clean environment, and a relatively low inflation rate. Suburban living in America represents a high degree of comfort unavailable in many other countries.

Despite the comfort of suburban life, for one who did not drive a car, I discovered that getting around was the most difficult challenge because public transportation was not easily available. Americans are so dependent on their cars that nothing seems to get done without them. A second challenge was the loneliness I experienced when the younger members of the family went to work. There were no children playing in the streets of the neighborhood as I was accustomed to seeing back in Asia. On occasion, I managed to catch a glimpse of the neighbors when they left or came back from work. We would wave to each other and exchange hello's without much time for socializing. The hustle and bustle seemed to leave everybody with little time. Confined mostly to the home, the telephone and television were my main connections to the outside world.

After the collapse of South Vietnam in 1975, more than a quarter million Vietnamese fled to the United States. Many settled in San Jose, California where I lived. To my utmost joy, I later found many of my former friends and acquaintances, including my next-door neighbor in Cholon for twenty years. It was much like a big family reunion. I did not feel lonely anymore now that I had so many old friends around.

The Enthusiasm Of My Students

A year or so after settling in California, I met the owner of a Chinese herb shop in Oakland who wanted me to join him as a resident physician. So, I resumed my private practice. A couple of years later, the owner of another herb shop in San Francisco asked me to join him. Thus, I found myself dividing my time between the two herb shops. As I slowly built up a clientele, my association and friendship with members of the local community also expanded.

Due to the low-tech and low-profile nature of Chinese medicine, the study and practice of this profession did not catch the enthusiasm of youths in China. During my career that spanned several decades, I met only a handful of young people who had expressed a sincere desire to learn Chinese medicine. Thus, I was pleasantly surprised when I discovered that there was a strong interest in Chinese medicine, especially in California where there were already a number of acupuncture schools offering licensure programs.

My private practice in San Francisco and Oakland facilitated contact with other local practitioners of Chinese medicine. Especially gratifying was the development of friendships with a large number of American-born acupuncturists and herbalists, some of whom when we met were in their late twenties. They had come to me with a burning desire to learn more about the application of Chinese herbs. We thus began a long and interesting dialogue covering both medical and cultural topics.

Our exchanges took on two approaches. Some became apprentices by coming to the herb shop for a day or two each week to observe how I diagnosed and prescribed herbs. Others organized seminars where I was invited to talk about certain medical cases and their treatment. These regular exchanges further deepened the understanding of Chinese medicine and our different cultures. Indeed, the enthusiasm of my American students encouraged me to write this book.

The Side Effects of Chemotherapy

One day, after I began practising in California, a Mr. Williams came to my office accompanied by his wife. He was in his mid-twenties, and appeared fragile in a six-foot frame. Williams was a computer engineer and loved basketball. He had had stomach trouble for a couple of years and the stomach pain haunted him occasionally. He obtained temporary relief by taking an ulcer medicine prescribed by his Western doctor.

During the past few months, Williams was experiencing frequent and intense stomach pain. A detailed checkup showed that it was cancer. Surgery was performed to remove the stomach. Williams left the hospital in less than three weeks, and resumed work one month later. Because the cancer had spread, he was receiving chemotherapy treatment.

The chemotherapy produced many adverse side effects. Since leaving the hospital, his body weight had dropped by almost one-third, and he had lost his hair. But the most unpleasant symptoms were nausea, loss of appetite, fatigue, and low spirits. Williams was referred to me by one of his friends.

Williams took my prescription regularly twice a week. The herbs did not interfere with his chemotherapy. As the chemicals eradicated the cancer, the herbs nourished the body, regulated and balanced the functions of the organs, and relieved the pain from the side effects of the chemotherapy.

Williams' condition improved visibly with an increase in appetite and body weight. "Your herbs really worked wonders!" was his comment. I was very happy to see a young man of another culture so ready to accept traditional medicine which he had not known about before. He continued to see me twice a month for half a year. Then unfortunately, the cancer could not be stopped. I paid him a visit during his last days. I was deeply touched when he held my hand and thanked me for bringing some happiness to the last months of his life.

AIDS: Can The Suffering Be Reduced?

The spread of AIDS has caused grave concern all over the world. Although the suffering of people dying of AIDS is no less than that of cancer patients, people seem to sympathize less with the former. The reasons are not difficult to understand. A large percentage of AIDS patients contract the disease through sharing drug needles, or engaging in unsafe sexual activities. Consequently, many people think of AIDS as someone else's problem rather than their own. Nevertheless, as a physician, I cannot bear to see the withering of an AIDS patient and the pain and indignity accompanying the disease.

Mr. Brown was a young man in his late twenties. He was confirmed to be HIV-positive, and was advised by the hospital to enroll in a monitoring and treatment program to delay the onset of full-blown AIDS. Brown was scared and depressed. He could not decide whether to enroll in the program. Some of his friends referred him to me. Both Brown and I did not harbor any false hope that Chinese medicine could cure AIDS. Brown knew that his days were numbered, but he feared the slow death and the Western method of treatment. He wanted to try an alternative medicine. I had to do what I could to lessen his suffering, and if possible, to delay the onset of AIDS.

Since no specific symptoms appear during the initial stage of HIV infection, I put Brown on a prescription of herbs that strengthened his body against infection. The herbs also increased his appetite, boosted his energy, and nourished his blood and skin. He saw me once a week and reported that he was feeling better overall. He was eating more, sleeping better, and enjoying the outdoors. This situation continued for almost two years during which Brown was able to avoid major infections, and had actually gained some weight. We were praying that the herbs would continue to postpone the onset of AIDS.

One day however, Brown came down with a fever. With a usually healthy individual, such fevers should disappear after two or three prescriptions. But Brown had the fever for more than a week. I suspected it was an AIDS symptom and persuaded Brown to seek Western treatment which could administer more potent drugs. Initially, Brown was reluctant to go because he knew from his friends that the treatment was as painful as the disease.

Tests at the hospital confirmed the arrival of AIDS. The doctors cured his fever, but Brown suffered from nausea and other side effects from the drugs treating the virus. Due to the breakdown of his immune system, Brown was plagued by one infection after another which caused fever, diarrhea, mouth sores, skin rashes, and bronchitis. Brown continued with the herbs in order to balance his body functions which had been disturbed by the powerful chemical drugs. I gave him a modified version of the prescription. Hardly a week went by when he was not affected by some kind of illness. However, Brown said that the herbs helped him a great deal in coping with his daily struggle.

After seven months, Brown eventually died as a result of pneumonia. I admired his courage during the last few months when he, despite being so afflicted, continued to visit me regularly. I only wished I could have done more to alleviate his suffering.

Skin Irritations

One day a Mrs. Li brought her ten-year-old son to see me. Due to itching, the boy could not stop scratching his knees and the surrounding area. The mother had been applying skin ointments for some time with little effect. Continuous scratching had already damaged the skin.

Another skin case involved a Mrs. Smith. She had had irritations on the face and the hands for a number of years. The skin of the affected areas were coarse, dry, and cracked. Medications and skin lotions that she had tried did not produce a permanent cure.

A third case involved a Vietnamese immigrant named Mrs. Tran who had ringworm. Small violet-red circles appeared on the abdomen and on some parts of the back. She was very uncomfortable because of the persistent itching. She had used various medications without significant results.

According to Chinese medicine, most skin conditions are related to the blood and the liver. Thus, herbal treatment consists of herbs that will "clean" the blood and "balance" the liver. A permanent cure normally takes a few months. During treatment, the patient must refrain from stimulating food and beverages such as pepper, vinegar, and alcohol. Sea food such as crab and shellfish may cause itching of the skin as well.

In the above cases, the patients came to see me once a week. Each time they reported some progress. I adjusted their prescriptions according to my observations and each patient's feedback. After a few months, all three experienced complete relief from the itching and their skin was restored to normal. In the case of Mrs. Tran, the ringworm sites changed slowly to violet, then to yellow, until they finally disappeared.

Fertility Is A Gift From Nature

Fertility is a gift from nature, and healthy persons reproduce without problems. However, many couples in America are not able to bear children for various reasons. Interestingly, infertility is seldom a problem for people in developing countries. One reason that so many American couples are affected by infertility is their postponement of having children. Then when they do decide, many are past their prime for producing children. Another reason is the use of the birth control pill which is designed to interfere with a woman's natural cycle of egg production and release by the ovaries. After several years of constant use, the body's natural reproductive cycle can be significantly altered. Even if the pill is discontinued, the longtime usage will most likely result in irregular menstruation. It may even produce a permanent negative impact on the fertility of the woman.

Infertility can also be caused by various physical problems that can reduce the chances of impregnation. In men, such problems can include lack of energy, difficulty in having or maintaining an erection, premature ejaculation, and low sperm count. In women, they can include anemia, irregular menstruation, and lack of energy, among others. For both men and women, herbs can help alleviate these physical problems.

In general, Chinese herbs restore the body to its normal balanced condition. In treating infertility, herbs are administered to eliminate the deficiencies that have caused infertility. For men, such herbs are aimed at increasing sperm production and restoring the vital energy of the kidneys. For women, the goal is strengthening the receptiveness of the reproductive organ toward sperm.

Two cases that I treated successfully were a Mr. Johnson and Mrs. Lyons. Mr. Johnson was in his mid-thirties. He was not in good health not because of illness, but because of persistent weakness in general. His face was pale, he was underweight, and was not at all active. His Western doctor had confirmed that he had a low sperm count. He took my prescription regularly for about a year, and gradually regained strength. His appetite improved and he put on more weight. He told me that he and his wife were enjoying having sex more often. Almost a year after he started on my prescription, he happily reported that his wife was pregnant with their first child.

Mrs. Lyons was an accountant in her early thirties. After four years of marriage, she and her lawyer husband finally wanted to have a child. The couple tried their best but could not bring about a pregnancy. (She had been on the pill for several years.) They came to see me and I determined that they had no major problems because they were in good health. All they needed were some herbs to increase the chances of pregnancy. I put the couple on separate fertility prescriptions for several months. They were cooperative patients, giving me feedback on what they felt after taking the formulas, so that I could adjust the prescription ingredients to further improve the effectiveness. About seven months after starting on the herbs, Mrs. Lyons was confirmed to be pregnant.

The Road To Longevity

The telephone rang one evening. A somewhat familiar voice asked if I remembered him. I took a couple of wild guesses. The caller then revealed his identity. It was Mu, my long-time friend and business partner in Cholon!

Mu did not leave Vietnam when the Saigon regime collapsed in 1975. Over the ensuing ten years, he lost his business and was sent to a labor camp in the countryside. Life was tougher than he could have possibly imagined. He was finally allowed to return to Cholon in 1986. Mu was a resilient man who never gave up. He rebuilt part of his former stationery business. Mu's enterprise slowly flourished, but he left for Canada anyway to join his daughters.

Having learned of my whereabouts, Mu made a special trip to San Francisco to see me. We were overjoyed when we met. After more than twenty years, Mu was as tough as ever, despite his grey hair and stooped back which he blamed on the hard labor of lifting stones in the Vietnamese countryside.

Mu's career had started as an employee in our herb store. His entrepreneurial talent carried him to eventual ownership of a million-dollar business of selling stationery products. Even though he lost his entire fortune, he was ready to forgive and never harbored bitterness toward anyone. He used to say: "Heaven gives and Heaven takes away, but a determined person will always find a way." This was what kept him going despite all the hardship after the Communist takeover. In his mid-seventies, five years my junior, he is still enthusiastic about the potential business opportunities in Cholon when the Hanoi government finally decides to open their domestic market to the world.

Mu is a survivor. He invested all his energy into building his dream business but seldom indulged in enjoying the fruits of his success. He donated generously to charity, believing that doing good to others would guarantee happiness in life. Mu liked to count his blessings. He did not see them as expanding deposit accounts in the bank. He found happiness in nurturing his children into independent adults. He took comfort in seeing the Buddhist temples he sponsored feed and shelter the poor. He enjoyed the company of friends, and was ready to offer help when he saw a need.

Mu realizes the fleeting nature of material wealth, as experienced by him personally. What one owns today can easily be swept away tomorrow by a natural disaster, or it can be destroyed by man-made events such as war. Even if one's material wealth can escape destruction, its departure from one's possession cannot be avoided. There exists only a thin line dividing life and death taking into account the occurrences of terminal disease, traffic accident and street crime. In between life and death, there also exists the possibility of incapacitation. All of these potential mishaps make life seem very fragile indeed.

If life seems so fragile and material wealth so fleeting, why are people so obsessed with materialism? Perhaps it is just part of human nature. However, many people have seen the light and discovered the true meaning of life. They amass material wealth, only to give it away to charity, or invest it in future generations. They realize that material things are only the means to an end, for everyone is born into this world empty-handed with no possessions, and has to surrender everything upon leaving. If we believe that life has a mission, it cannot be the creation of material wealth because we shall lose it all at the time of death. What makes ownership of material things meaningful during one's lifetime is the good deeds one does with them in this world. This sounds simple and true, yet so difficult to appreciate, let alone to practise.

If good deeds and happiness are the meaning of life, longevity will no longer take on any significance. It is better to live twenty years in happiness by doing good to others, than to live forty years in misery without seeing the true meaning of life. Consequently, longevity is mainly a state of mind and should not be measured in years.

I am fortunate to have Mu as a close friend and to share his philosophy about life. I have noticed that people who hold similar beliefs as Mu manage to live longer. The reason is that they are happier. They are able to throw away their obsession with expanding or losing their material wealth. Obsession breeds worry and anxiety, which have a debilitating effect on one's health especially when these emotions plague a person day after day.

Understanding the meaning of life is already halfway toward achieving longevity. Taking care of one's health is the other part. The key to good health is prevention, which consists of two aspects that must be pursued in parallel. The first is the realization that humans are an integral part of nature. As such, we must learn to respect and live in harmony with nature. Polluting and upsetting the delicate balance of nature can only create misery for mankind. The second aspect is the practice of moderation. This means maintaining a balance between work, play, eating, rest, and exercise. It also means maintaining a healthy and balanced diet, and protecting the body against infection.

As a practitioner, I have been exposed to a great variety of infections. However, by taking good care of myself, I have seldom been overcome by an illness. I practise prevention everyday by maintaining a balance in my activities. For exercise, many of my patients think that I practise Kung Fu, Qi Gong, or Tai Chi. But in actuality, I just walk two miles everyday in my neighborhood.

An additional aspect of prevention is the centuries-old Chinese tradition of incorporating herbs and foods that can help prevent disease, into the daily meals. How this is done varies with the geographic regions of China. Since I am from Canton, the herbs and foods that I use will reflect the traditions of southern China. (See chapter 8 for a discussion of preventing illness using herbs and special foods. In addition, see chapter 7 for a formula for longevity.)

How Costly Is The Automobile?

For a first-time visitor to America, a lasting impression is the multi-lane highway full of automobiles, mostly with just one person per car. America's love affair with the automobile continues to grow and grow. Besides its utility and convenience, the automobile provides an expression of traditional American values such as freedom, independence, and individualism. While private car ownership is a luxury for most countries, the car has become almost an absolute necessity in American life. The car has transformed our society and way of life more than any other invention in history.

From a health standpoint, more driving means less walking, which in turn means deprivation of the most basic exercise that is part of daily life. In addition, driving can be stressful because of the constant sitting and of having to focus close attention on the road. As the stress adds up, one's physical and mental well-being are affected. This is certainly reflected in the incivility that occurs on the road every day. Interestingly, once out of the car, people behave more gently toward one another. Hence, the automobile brings out the worst in people probably because of the stress caused by driving.

In addition, the cost of the automobile to the environment is multiplying precipitously, as evidenced by the polluted air, and mountains of rubber tires, and other discarded auto parts. Americans are proud of their car ownership statistics which average two cars per family. This sets an example for the rest of the world to follow, for they want to attain this standard of living, too. If private car ownership continues to grow, especially in the developing countries which account for most of the world's population, what will happen to the environment decades from now?

Low-Cost Health Care For Society

Health care is the most important among all consumer services. The demand for health care is universal. The need increases with age as the physical condition of a person weakens. When a person must see a doctor or take a prescription, it is due to a physical or emotional condition that forces that person to seek help. Consequently, charging a high price for medical help when a person is in distress is not only cruel, but immoral.

Health care is a moral issue if we believe in love and care for ourselves and other people. It is also a good investment because better health improves productivity and lessens the burden to society. There is no question that health care should be made available to all. The problem is how and to what extent. It is the responsibility of a society and its government to find a standard that is both universal and affordable. Achieving that standard ultimately depends on the success of cost containment for medical services.

In Asian societies where traditional Chinese medicine is widely practised, a patient can get help easily without the need for government subsidy. Although a small consultation fee is charged, the practitioner with a kind heart is always willing to waive the fee for those who cannot afford to pay. During my thirty years of practice in Cholon, I dedicated one afternoon of the week to free consultation for the poor.

Furthermore, traditional herbs are quite inexpensive, and their cost is stable despite periodic bad weather, war, and political turmoil in the places of origin. Because many herbs have overlapping healing effects, the herbalist can always substitute high-price herbs with cheaper ones, thus sparing the patient's budget. Apart from what the herbalist can do, the owner of the herb shop is inclined to waive the charge for the herbs if the patient is in a dire financial strait.

The hospitals that provide traditional medical services in Asia are either run by government or charity organizations. Hospital expenses are low because of low staff cost, and the absence of high-tech equipment. In China for example, health care is even brought to the remote villages by traveling doctors. Thus, in Asia where the standards of living and medical technology are relatively low, health care costs are easily contained. Although the quality cannot match that of the West, health care is maintained at an appropriate level consistent with the local standard of living, and is acceptable to the local population. Apart from low-cost traditional medicine which is available to all, Western medicine is also accessible for those who can afford it. Some hospitals of Western medicine base their services on the complexity of diseases they treat, and are also subsidized by the government. In China today, Chinese and Western medicines are integrated in many hospitals in order to reap the benefits of both modalities.

In America, the health care system is quite different. The standard of living is high, the medical field is highly technologized and specialized, and the health care system is extremely sophisticated and includes the participation of insurance companies and attorneys. The consequence is a high price for patients, and high cost for employers, government, and even for practitioners. The problem we must face is cost containment, because an increasing number of consumers and employers cannot afford to pay for health care. The government is also finding it difficult to fund a rapidly increasing health care subsidy. Another problem is the quality of care. Universal coverage seems out of reach, and increasingly limited coverage becomes the rule, especially for the elderly.

While we continue to grapple with cost containment, it may be worthwhile to investigate the possibility of incorporating traditional methods of health care into the American system. The low-cost nature of Chinese medicine presents a great advantage. The effectiveness of Chinese herbs for common illnesses can vastly reduce the claim on existing health care resources. Since Chinese medicine emphasizes prevention, especially through the use of tonic herbs which invigorate the body and boost its defenses, an additional savings can be achieved. Another advantage of Chinese medicine is that patients receive customized herbal prescriptions that are inexpensive and more desirable than pharmaceuticals which are only for the "average" patient, and which usually cause side effects. Thus, many benefits can be derived by adopting traditional Chinese medicine as an adjunct to Western medicine in America.

God Bless America, My Adopted Country

One morning in the spring of 1985, my son John, his wife, and I were sitting in a large room of the U.S. Immigration Office in San Jose, California, for the naturalization swear-in ceremony. There were two hundred or so citizens-to-be, mainly of Asian and Mexican descent. The judge came in, performed the short but solemn ceremony, then congratulated and welcomed us as citizens of the United States.

At age seventy-five, this was to be my third and last citizenship. I was born a Chinese citizen but saw my native country go through turbulent and agonizing times. When I was young, Chinese citizenship carried almost no rights and privileges compared to those enjoyed by the foreign occupiers on Chinese soil. In my middle age, I became a South Vietnamese citizen but lost my citizenship as the country fell apart twenty years later. Now, I am happy to have found an adopting country. I am proud to be an American.

The greatness of America lies in the high principles and ideals expressed in the Declaration of Independence and safeguarded by the Constitution. The democratic system, the free enterprise spirit, and the resultant opportunities available have attracted a constant stream of immigrants from all over the world. America's ready acceptance and toleration of many things foreign infuse the country with new ideas and energy so essential for self-renewal. America is a relatively young country whose people believe in dreams and view things with a certain degree of naivete. This is a unique American quality. It is desirable because only great dreams can lead to great achievements previously thought to be impossible.

With the collapse of the Soviet Union and the rising economic power of Europe and Pacific Asia, the world is evolving into a multipolar system where economic competition will intensify to an extent never seen before. As other countries develop, the importance of the U.S. economy relative to the rest of the world will undoubtedly decline. As a consequence, American influence in world affairs will be more limited. As the twenty-first century approaches, America is immersed in enormous domestic problems such as the rising cost of health care, the federal deficit, difficulty in job creation, declining standard of education which in turn lowers productivity, drug abuse, increasing street violence, and the breakup of the family unit.

The next century will be one when the rest of the world will be watching closely how we Americans try to transform and reinvent ourselves. Our domestic problems will tax every bit of our resolve, ingenuity, and courage. Our ability to lead the world will depend on the success of our domestic reforms. As always, great countries achieve great things through the willingness to accept the challenges posed by great problems. As a nation, we have shown the world that we are able to gather our strength and resources to tackle the great problems facing us. We may stumble or fail as we have done in the past. However, we shall learn and recover in the process. We are sure that we shall triumph in the end.

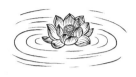

Chapter 7

Herbal Prescriptions

The Art Of Writing An Effective Prescription

The primary goal of the medical profession is to alleviate human suffering due to illness. For an herbalist, writing an effective prescription is what the job is all about. To bring about an herbal cure is by no means a mechanical procedure governed by a fixed set of formulas. Through trial and error early in the herbalist's career, success eventually comes when enough experience about and insight into a diversity of medical cases have been gained. The factors contributing to the complexity of formulating an effective prescription are enumerated below.

First, most herbs have multiple healing effects. The herbalist normally wants to enhance only some desired effects and suppress the rest. This is done through combination with other herbs. But the other herbs in the formula also have multiple effects. Thus, the method of correctly combining herbs to yield the desired effect is probably the most difficult skill to master. This will be explained later in this chapter.

Second, every patient is unique in body chemistry and physical condition. An herbal prescription that works for one person may not work for another.

Third, the herbalist depends on the patient for a second visit to examine the results of the first prescription. In difficult cases, more consultations may be required to enable the herbalist to complete the cure with a better prescription. If the patient does not return, the herbalist will be deprived of valuable feedback.

Fourth, each herbal prescription is unique for each patient. If the prescription does not work, the herbalist shoulders all the blame and must formulate a better one. This is in contrast to synthetic drugs. For example, if aspirin does not work for a particular patient, the physician simply switches to another ready-made drug and informs the patient of the unsuitability of aspirin for that particular case.

Where should one begin in order to become an herbalist? The logical starting point is to amass the knowledge about different herbs and their therapeutic effects. This was done by apprenticeship in the old times. However, beginning in the 1930s, a structured program of Chinese herbal medicine has been offered by medical schools in China. Similar programs are also offered by schools of acupuncture and oriental medicine elsewhere. The knowledge of herbs consists of empirical evidence of their healing effects as recorded in medical literature. Thus, would-be herbalists can learn the basic technique for writing prescriptions at school and from textbooks. This knowledge serves as a foundation for the training and internship period when supervised treatment of patients occurs. The final test comes in the real world when practising herbalists must deal with patients on their own. This is where the road to mastery begins.

Today, there are around one thousand herbs that are commercially available. This represents the universe of herbs from which an herbalist can prescribe. Some are rare and others are very expensive. Since many herbs have overlapping effects, based on experience, the herbalist can narrow this universe of herbs to around three hundred of the less expensive ones. Generally, these include the herbalist's own favored herbs from which he/she normally prescribes. I usually write a prescription that consists of ten to fifteen herbs. Other herbalists have their own unique styles and methods of cure. Given this diversity of prescription styles, therapeutic effects can vary widely. The ultimate test is determined by the healing progress of the patient.

In Chinese medicine, there can be more than one way to treat an illness. In writing an herbal prescription, there is no standard procedure to follow, except for some basic formulas presented in the classical medical literature. Thus, the herbalist has the sole responsibility of delivering an effective prescription. If other factors remain the same, the herbalist who is more experienced and has seen a diversity of cases is in a better position to heal an ailment. Writing an herbal prescription is more of an art than a science. Like music and painting, one perfects the art simply by doing it everyday. Just following a textbook can never make a Beethoven or a Picasso. Mastery comes with small refinements over many years of practice and reflection. The few years spent in school provide only a foundation to serve as a starting point.

To treat an ailment, the traditional herbalist first diagnoses by observation, touch, smell, by feeling the pulse on the wrist, and by asking questions. No modern diagnostic techniques are employed such as X-rays or blood tests. The herbalist then comes to a conclusion as to what type of ailment it is and what herbs to prescribe. Starting with the basic herbs learned in school, the herbalist adds to and subtracts from this basic list according to the particular condition of the patient. The herbalist then determines the proportions of each herb that will yield the best possible effect.*
The patient takes the prescription to an herb store, where the herbs

*Herbal formulas that have already been prepared in pill form may also be selected.

will be put together in the prescribed quantities in a package. The patient takes the package home, boils it in water for about an hour to make a tea which the patient then drinks.

With regard to diagnosis, the question that arises is, what are the chances of misdiagnosis when no sophisticated equipment is used? A diagnosis is a human judgment based on the facts obtained. These facts can be obtained through a variety of methods, both traditional and modern. In some instances, modern methods are more effective, and in others, traditional diagnosis is sufficient to yield a correct conclusion about the disease. This does not mean that traditional methods cannot be supplemented by modern ones as human knowledge expands, or that the use of modern technology necessarily leads to a correct diagnosis.

Some may question the risks involved when very little laboratory analyses and controlled clinical tests on herbs have been done. In actuality, millions of people around the world, especially in Asia, have been using herbs since time immemorial. That herbs are still widely used is testimony to their safety and effectiveness. Herbs are products of nature which nourish and sustain life. If we consider ourselves a part of nature, we will appreciate the value of nature's products, and will not hesitate to take advantage of these products.

The effects of herbs contrast greatly with those of synthetic drugs. Herbs usually do not produce an immediate cure. Their effects can take hours or even days to be manifested. When they cure an illness, they also bring the body to a better overall condition. In contrast, synthetic drugs are invented to cure very specific ailments through concentrated dosages. Unlike natural herbs, they do not have a long history of empirical testing on a diversity of subjects. To compensate for this, synthetic drugs must rely on rigorous laboratory and clinical testing to establish their safety and effectiveness. Even with all the testing, most pharmaceuticals still produce side effects.

To write an effective prescription, the herbalist should stress the therapeutic effects of herbs more than medical theory. It is better to rely on hard facts than on a human concept that is constantly undergoing refinement. During my sixty years of medical practice, I have always let empirical knowledge and practical experience be the foundation of my prescriptions. The first prescription I write for a patient is mainly based on my diagnosis. This first prescription seldom produces a complete cure. The patient's second visit (and ensuing visits if necessary) is when I practice the art of prescription writing. At this time, the results of the previously prescribed herbs can be closely examined and evaluated. Furthermore, the results will validate my previous prescription and diagnosis. Based on this additional information, I can gain more insight into the particular case, and adjust the prescription for a complete cure.

The Composition of the Herbal Prescription

As mentioned above, combining herbs in a prescription to deliver an effective cure is a complex and intricate art that can only be learned through practice. There are no straightforward rules about how herbs should be combined. The composition of a formula depends on the condition of the patient and the style of the herbalist. To help illustrate this point, the following table is presented.

Strengthening Effects of Selected Herbs on the Body

	Heart	Liver	Stomach	Lungs	Kidneys	Blood	Qi/Energy
Ginseng (ren shen)	•		•				•
Tang-kuei (dang gui)	•	•				•	
Peony root bark (mu dan pi)	•	•			•	•	
Notoginseng (san qi)		•	•			•	
Astragalus (huang qi)				•			•
Psoralea (bu gu zhi)					•		•
Poria (fu ling)	•		•	•			
Atractylodes (bai zhu)			•				•
Ophiopogon (mai men dong)	•		•	•			
Ligusticum (chuan xiong)	•	•				•	
Biota seed (bai zi ren)	•	•			•		
Polygala (yuan zhi)	•			•	•		
Lycium fruit (gou qi zi)		•			•		
Peony (bai shao)		•				•	
Gentiana (long dan cao)		•	•				
Raw rehmannia (sheng di huang)		•				•	•
Ash bark (qin pi)		•	•				
Saussurea (mu xiang)		•	•				
Hawthorn fruit (shan zha)		•	•				
Cynanchum (bai qian)			•				•

	Heart	Liver	Stomach	Lungs	Kidneys	Blood	Qi/Energy
Strengthening Effects of Selected Herbs on the Body (continued)							
Brassica seed (*bai jie zi*)		•	•	•			
Agrimony (*xian he cao*)		•		•			
Gecko (*ge jie*)				•	•		
Eucommia (*du zhong*)		•			•		
Morinda (*ba ji tian*)		•			•		
Dodder seed (*tu si zi*)		•			•		
Cynamorium (*suo yang*)		•			•		

The herbs in the table represent a sample of my favorite herbs; each has strengthening capabilities on various parts of the body. Based on this table, it is easy to identify the appropriate herbs to be used for an ailment associated with an organ. Suppose a kidney ailment is to be treated, the herbalist can check the "kidneys" column to find all the herbs listed in that column. These, then, are the herbs that can be included in the prescription package for they have a common strengthening effect on the kidneys.

However, the multiple effects of those herbs warrant further thought. This is where the diagnosis and the insight come in. Does the patient have a weak heart? Does the patient complain about poor appetite? Does the kidney ailment lower the patient's energy level significantly? Is there a fever accompanying the kidney ailment? What will be the body's reactions to those herbs? There may be other observations and considerations to take into account. The following discussion should help elucidate this line of thinking.

Moutan (*mu dan pi*). Besides strengthening the kidneys, this herb also strengthens the heart, the liver and the blood. According to the Five Phases correspondences (see chapter 1), weak kidneys will lead to a weak liver (generating sequence) but a strong heart (restraining sequence). It should be noted that "strong" and "weak" are only relative in meaning because we are referring to the balance and harmony of body functions. Consequently, this herb has a desirable side effect on the liver but not on the heart. However, if the patient has a weak heart as manifested by a weak pulse, strengthening the heart will be desirable and will not be of concern. If the patient has a strong pulse but weak kidneys, this herb may not be suitable due to the side effect on the heart. This herb's nourishing effect on the blood is considered desirable.

Psoralea *(bu gu zhi)*. The only other effect this herb has is increasing the energy level, which is desirable.

Biota seed *(bai zi ren)*. The same reasoning can be applied as for peony root bark *(mu dan pi)*.

Polygala *(yuan zhi)*. In addition to the kidneys, this herb strengthens the heart and the lungs. The effect on the heart may be of concern as explained for peony root bark *(mu dan pi)*. However, the effect on the lungs indirectly helps the kidneys (generating sequence). Thus, this herb gives the kidneys an additional boost.

Lycium fruit *(gou qi zi)*. This herb strengthens both the kidneys and the liver. Strengthening the kidneys also has a positive effect on the liver (generating sequence).

Gecko *(ge jie)*. This herb strengthens both the kidneys and the lungs. Strengthening the lungs indirectly helps the kidneys (generating sequence).

For the remaining herbs which include eucommia *(du zhong)*, morinda *(ba ji tian)*, dodder seed *(tu si zi)*, and cynamorium *(suo yang)*, the same reasoning applies as for lycium fruit *(gou qi zi)*.

Based on the above thinking, all ten herbs identified can be included in the prescription package. These herbs will reinforce each other when they act on the kidneys. In addition, they will affect the heart, liver, lungs, blood, and energy level. But these effects will be moderate relative to the reinforced effect on the kidneys. With regard to the three herbs that also strengthen the heart, if the patient has a weak heart, then the effect of the herbs will be a positive one. If the heart is not weak, these three herbs can still be used because as the kidneys are strengthened, the heart is also restrained. Depending on the patient's other symptoms, herbs can be substituted or added to yield the desired effects.

For a prescription to be effective, it must include several herbs so that they will reinforce each other. A formula must be able to achieve two things: a main effect to cure the ailment, and a supportive effect that will not disrupt the body functions but will bring the body to a higher level of balanced strength.

The remainder of this chapter presents prescriptions for common ailments. The herbs and formulas are ones that I have used over the past decades. Each of these prescriptions serves as a guide only. It does not list proportions or weights, which must be determined for each individual case. By studying these formulas, readers will gain more insight into the art of prescription writing. In addition since herbalists and herb supplies are not available to every patient who needs them, I have prepared herbal prescriptions in tablet form. They are available from Health Concerns (see resource section).

AIDS Relief

At this time, there is no known medicine that can cure the dreadful disease of AIDS. The AIDS patient is subject to all kinds of infection as the body loses its defense against diseases.

Prescription Rationale

Many Chinese herbs are capable of improving the overall condition of the body. This prescription is not aimed at addressing a specific infection. Instead, its intention is to nourish the blood, reinvigorate the vital energy, and to restore the equilibrium of the body functions so that its defense mechanism is able to fight infections.

Recommended Herbs

English Name	Pharmaceutical Name	Chinese Name
Tang-kuei	Radix Angelicae Sinensis	*dang gui*
Ligusticum	Radix Ligustici Chuanxiong	*chuan xiong*
Codonopsis	Radix Codonopsitis Pilosulae	*dang shen*
Rehmannia	Radix Rehmanniae Glutinosae Conquitae	*shu di huang*
Cistanche	Herba Cistanches Deserticolae	*rou cong rong*
Atractylodes	Rhizoma Atractylodis Macrocephalae	*bai zhu*
Cinnamon twig	Ramulus Cinnamomi Cassiae	*gui zhi*
Morinda	Radix Morindae Officinalis	*ba ji tian*
Peony	Radix Paeoniae Lactiflorae	*bai shao*
Cynomorium	Herba Cynomorii Songarici	*suo yang*

Alcohol Poisoning

Excessive alcohol consumption over a long period can have a devastating effect on one's health. For the occasional drinker, overindulging can aggravate an existing health problem.

Prescription Rationale

This prescription is intended for occasional drinkers who experience a bout of alcohol poisoning. The following herbs "clean" the blood, restore the vitality of the liver and kidneys, and regulate the water content of the body.

Recommended Herbs

English Name	Pharmaceutical Name	Chinese Name
American ginseng	Radix Panacis Quinquefolii	xi yang shen
Pueraria flower	Flos Pperariae	ge hua
Viola	Herba cum Radice Violae Yedoensitis	zi hua di ding
Chaenomelis	Fructus Chaenomelis	mu gua
Licorice	Radix Glycyrrhizae Uralensis	gan cao
Raw rehmannia	Radix Rehmanniae Glutinosae	sheng di huang
Curcuma	Tuber Curcumae	yu jin
Magnolia bark	Cortex Magnoliae Officinalis	hou po
Jasmine flower	Flos Jasmini Officinale	su xin hua

Allergy To Pollen

Allergy to pollen, or hayfever, is a common condition, especially during the spring. Symptoms may include sneezing, coughing, nasal congestion, watery eyes, and skin rash.

Prescription Rationale

The following herbs are intended to relieve itching; to reduce swelling; to strengthen the lungs; and to nourish the skin, the eyes and other sense organs. The herbs also have an overall effect of promoting the flow of vital energy.

Recommended Herbs

English Name	Pharmaceutical Name	Chinese Name
Siler	Radix Ledebouriellae Divaricatae	*fang feng*
Xanthium fruit	Fructus Xanthii Sibirici	*cang er zi*
Perilla leaf	Folium Perillae Frutescentis	*zi su ye*
Cinnamon twig	Ramulus Cinnamomi Cassiae	*gui zhi*
Atractylodes	Rhizoma Atractylodis	*cang zhu*
Codonopsis	Radix Codonopsitis Pilosulae	*dang shen*
Angelica root	Radix Angelicae Dahuricae	*bai zhi*
Honeylocust spine	Spina Gleditsiae Sinensis	*zao jiao ci*
Bupleurum	Radix Bupleuri	*chai hu*
Lonicera flower	Flos Lonicerae Japonicae	*jin yin hua*

Appendicitis

Inflammation of the appendix is sometimes due to blockage of the appendix opening by a small stone formed from digestive wastes. Chinese herbs are effective during the initial stages of appendicitis. However, infection and gangrene may lead to bursting of the appendix wall which requires surgery to remove the appendix and to clean the abdominal cavity.

Prescription Rationale

According to Chinese medicine, appendix inflammation is due to malfunction of the vital organs, especially the digestive system, which results in food stagnation or sluggishness of the intestines. The herbs in the formula below are used to reduce inflammation and pain, and to clean the blood. In addition, the herbs invigorate the digestive system so that food stagnation is eliminated.

Recommended Herbs

English Name	Pharmaceutical Name	Chinese Name
Tang-kuei	Radix Angelicae Sinensis	*dang gui*
Gardenia fruit	Fructus Gardeniae Jasminoidis	*zhi zi*
Scutellaria	Radix Scutellariae Baicalensis	*huang qin*
Akebia	Caulis Mutong	*mu tong*
Notoginseng	Radix Notoginseng	*san qi*
Coptis	Rhizoma Coptidis	*huang lian*
Phellodendron	Cortex Phellodendri	*huang bai*
Peach seed	Semen Persicae	*tao ren*
Pueraria	Radix Puerariae	*ge gen*
Raw rehmannia	Radix Rehmanniae Glutinosae	*sheng di huang*
Saussurea	Radix Aucklandiae Lappae	*mu xiang*
Bupleurum	Radix Bupleuri	*chai hu*

Arthritis

Inflammation of the joints, known as arthritis, is due to various factors. Presently, there is no known medicine that can cure arthritis. The ailment tends to worsen with aging or with sudden weather changes. In Chinese medicine, arthritis is known as "wind damp" illness, due to the fact that the aches and pains of the joints worsen after an individual is exposed to cold, wind, or dampness/humimidty.

Prescription Rationale

From the Chinese medical viewpoint, exposure to cold, wind, or dampness changes the nature of the blood to a certain extent. As a consequence, blood flow becomes sluggish. Dampness is thought to be captured in the tissues around the joints, and cannot be "flushed out" by the slowed blood flow. Relief lies in restoring the nature of the blood to its original state, thus alleviating the aches and pains of the joints. The following prescription produces two effects: reinvigorating the blood flow and reducing arthritis inflammation.

Arthritis, *continued*

Recommended Herbs

English Name	Pharmaceutical Name	Chinese Name
Tang-kuei	Radix Angelicae Sinensis	*dang gui*
Kirin ginseng	Radix Ginseng	*ji lin shen*
Chinese quince	Fructus Chaenomelis	*mu gua*
Cinnamon twig	Ramulus Cinnamomi Cassiae	*gui zhi*
Rehmannia	Radix Rehmanniae Glutinosae Conquitae	*shu di huang*
Millettia	Radix et Caulis Jixueteng	*ji xue teng*
Fleeceflower root	Radix Polygoni Multiflori	*he shou wu*
Cistanche	Herba Cistanches Deserticolae	*rou cong rong*
Loranthus	Ramulus Sangjisheng	*sang ji sheng*
Pubescent root	Radix Angelicae Pubescentis	*du huo*
Notoginseng	Radix Notoginseng	*san qi*
Wild ginger	Herba cum Radix Asari	*xi xin*
Achyranthes	Radix Achyranthis Bidentatae	*niu xi*

Prevention

Protect the body against sudden changes of weather
Avoid long periods of exposure to cold, wind, or dampness
Avoid overexertion
Rest sufficiently
Avoid alcoholic beverages

Asthma

Asthma is characterized by shortness of breath, wheezing, coughing, and gasping, due to constriction of the bronchi. An asthma attack may be triggered by an allergy such as to pollen, dust, dander, and the like. Respiratory infections, exposure to cold air or to smoke can also set off attacks as can physical or emotional stress.

Prescription Rationale

The following prescription is aimed at reducing cough and other asthma symptoms. The herbs help nourish the lungs and the respiratory tract, promote blood circulation, and dispel harmful factors of Cold and Wind in the body.

Recommended Herbs

English Name	Pharmaceutical Name	Chinese Name
Ephedra	Herba Ephedrae	*ma huang*
Siler	Radix Ledbouriellae Divaricatae	*fang feng*
Gypsum	Gypsum	*shi gao*
Gardenia fruit	Fructus Gardeniae Jasminoidis	*zhi zi*
Apricot seed	Semen Armeniacae Pruni	*xing ren*
Wild ginger	Herba cum Radix Asari	*xi xin*
Licorice	Radix Glycyrrhizae Uralensis	*gan cao*
Pinellia	Rhizoma Pinelliae Ternatae	*ban xia*
Fritillaria	Bulbus Fritillariae Cirrhosae	*chuan bei mu*
Cinnamon twig	Ramulus Cinnamomi Cassiae	*gui zhi*

Prevention

Avoid ice-cold and peppery foods
Avoid environmental conditions that can trigger an asthma attack

Baldness

Baldness, especially in men as they age, is usually hereditary, and should not be considered an illness.

Prescription Rationale

Chinese medical theory considers the hair an extension of the blood. Thus, nourishing the blood should produce healthy hair. The herbs in the following formula are used to maintain healthy hair, promote hair growth, and delay the onset of baldness.

Recommended Herbs

English Name	Pharmaceutical Name	Chinese Name
Tang-kuei	Radix Angelica Sinensis	*dang gui*
Lycium fruit	Fructus Lycii	*gou qi zi*
Codonopsis	Radix Codonopsitis Pilosulae	*dang shen*
Cistanche	Herba Cistanches Deserticolae	*rou cong rong*
Ho shou wu	Radix Polygoni Multiflori	*he shou wu*
Rehmannia	Radix Rehmanniae Glutinosae Conquitae	*shu di huang*
Ligusticum	Radix Ligustici Chuanxiong	*chuan xiong*
Red peony	Radix Paeoniae Rubrae	*chi shao*
Ligustrum	Fructus Ligustri Lucidi	*nu zhen zi*
Cornus	Fructus Corni Officinalis	*shan zhu yu*
Gelatin	Gelatinum Corii Asini	*e jiao*

Beauty Enhancement For Women

Beauty is composed of two aspects : natural and artificial. Natural beauty is reflected by the individual's physical and emotional states. Artificial beauty is the individual's appeareance which can be enhanced through cosmetics, apparel, or even plastic surgery.

Prescription Rationale

A woman's natural beauty such as her deportment, composure, and behavior is simply a manifestation of the state of her health. Chinese herbs can enhance natural beauty by improving the woman's overall physical and emotional conditions. The following prescription emphasizes nourishing the blood, moistening the skin, and harmonizing the functions of vital organs.

Recommended Herbs

English Name	Pharmaceutical Name	Chinese Name
Aster root	Radix Asteris Tatarici	*zi wan*
Eclipta	Herba Ecliptae Prostratae	*han lian cao*
Viola	Herba cum Radice Violae Yedoensitis	*zi hua di ding*
American ginseng	Radix Panacis Quinguefolii	*xi yang shen*
Lonicera flower	Flos Lonicerae Japonicae	*jin yin hua*
Jasmine flower	Flos Jasmini Officinale	*su xin hua*
Rose flower	Flos Rosae Rugosae	*mei gui hua*
Raw rehmannia	Radix Rehmanniae Glutinosae	*sheng di huang*
Ligustrum	Fructus Ligusri Lucidi	*nu zhen zi*
Abrus	Herba Abri Fruticulosis	*ji gu cao*
Bupleurum	Radix Bupleuri	*chai hu*
Cassia seed	Semen Cassiae	*jue ming zi*
Peony	Radix Paeoniae Lactiflorae	*bai shao*
Licorice	Radix Glycyrrhizae Uralensis	*gan cao*

Brittle Bones

With aging, the bones gradually lose their density. Weakened bones usually lead to lack of strength in the back, arms, and legs. The bones are also prone to fracture, thus care should be taken to avoid falling or over-exertion.

Prescription Rationale

The onset of brittle bones can be delayed by taking herbs that enhance the overall vitality of the body. Such herbs compose the following formula which nourishes the blood, strengthens the bones and increases the collagen content, removes the harmful factors of Wind and Dampness in the body, and harmonizes the functions of the organs.

Recommended Herbs

English Name	Pharmaceutical Name	Chinese Name
Tang-kuei	Radix Angelicae Sinensis	*dang gui*
Rehmannia	Radix Rehmanniae Glutinosae Conquitae	*shu di huang*
Ligusticum	Radix Ligustici Chuanxiong	*chuan xiong*
Red peony	Radix Paeoniae Rubrae	*chi shao*
Ardisia	Radix Ardisiae Gigantifoliae	*zou ma tai*
Tortoise plastron	Plastrum Testudinis	*gui ban*
Deer tendon	Tendo Cervi	*lu jin*
Tortoise plastron gelatin	Gelatinum Plastri Testudinis	*gui ban jiao*
Chinese quince	Fructus Chaenomelis	*mu gua*
Millettia	Radix et Caulis Jixueteng	*ji xue teng*
Evodia	Fructus Evodiae Rutaecarpae	*wu zhu yu*
Cinnamon twig	Ramulus Cinnamomi Cassiae	*gui zhi*
Codonopsis	Radix Codonopsitis Pilosulae	*dang shen*
Licorice	Radix Glycyrrhizae Uralensis	*gan cao*

Brittle Bones, *continued*

Prevention

Maintain a balanced diet
Eat foods that have high calcium and gelatin contents
Exercise regularly
For the elderly, avoid over-exertion and situations that may precipitate a fall

Chemotherapy Side Effects

The adverse side effects from chemotherapy treatment include nausea, loss of appetite, weight loss, and loss of hair, among others.

Prescription Rationale

The strong chemicals used during chemotherapy can disturb the intricate balance of body functions. The following prescription is aimed at tonifying the organs and nourishing the blood, thus enabling the patient to feel better and to cope with the undesirable side effects.

Recommended Herbs

English Name	Pharmaceutical Name	Chinese Name
Tang-kuei	Radix Angelica Sinensis	*dang gui*
Codonopsis	Radix Codonopsitis Pilosulae	*dang shen*
Cornus	Fructus Corni Officinalis	*shan zhu yu*
Raw rehmannia	Radix Rehmanniae Glutinosae	*sheng di huang*
Peony root	Radix Paeoniae Lactiflorae	*bai shao*
Astragalus	Radix Astragali Membranacei	*huang qi*
Mulberry	Fructus Mori Albae	*sang shen*
Eucommia	Cortex Eucommiae Ulmoidis	*du zhong*
Chinese yam	Rhizoma Dioscoreae Oppositae	*shan yao*
Melia	Fructus Meliae Toosendan	*chuan lian zi*
Polygonatum	Rhizhoma Polygonati Odorati	*yu zhu*
Polygala	Radix Polygalae Tenuifoliae	*yuan zhi*
Eclipta	Herba Ecliptae Prostratae	*han lian cao*

Children's Common Ailments

Children under ten years of age become ill often due to the following reasons : a sudden weather change, food inappropriate for their sensitive digestive systems, and exposure to infections. Pediatric illnesses include fever, cough, diarrhea, ear pain, sore throat, phlegm, vomiting, indigestion, among others.

Prescription Rationale

When treating children with herbs, the formula should be gentle yet effective. The goal of the following formula is to reduce fever or excess body heat, cleanse the digestive system, moisten the lungs and clear the respiratory tract, and resolve phlegm.

Recommended Herbs

English Name	Pharmaceutical Name	Chinese Name
Forsythia fruit	Fructus Forsythiae Suspensae	*lian qiao*
Chrysanthemum	Flos Chrysanthemi Morifolii	*ju hua*
Peppermint	Herba Menthae Haplocalycis	*bo he*
Peucedanum	Radix Peucidani	*qian hu*
Eupatorium	Herba Eupatorii Fortunei	*pei lan*
Medicated leaven	Massa Fermentata	*shen qu*
Immature orange	Fructus Immaturus Aurantii Citri	*zhi shi*
Mulberry leaf	Folium Mori Albae	*sang ye*
Platycodon	Radix Platycodi Grandiflori	*jie geng*
Loquat leaf	Folium Eriobotryae Japonicae	*pi pa ye*
Trichosanthes peel	Pericarpium Trichosanthis	*gua lou pi*
Fritillaria	Bulbus Fritillariae Thunbergii	*zhe bei mu*
Pinellia	Rhizoma Pinelliae Ternatae	*ban xia*

Children's Common Ailments, *continued*

Prevention

Protect the child from sudden change in weather conditions

Do not overfeed

Make sure foods are clean and unspoiled before feeding

Know the child's sensitivities to various foods

Avoid exposing the child to environments where there is poor sanitation or contagious diseases

Constipation

Constipation is primarily caused by three factors. The first is diet imbalance. A diet that lacks fiber and water will likely bring about constipation. Foods that increase heat in the body can also cause constipation (see chapter 4). The second factor has to do with one's profession. Many jobs confine people to chairs for many hours a day. Long periods of sitting without movement can bring about constipation. The third factor is due to fever that consumes water in the body. In this case, constipation is only a side effect of the illness. When the fever is cured, constipation will usually resolve spontaneously.

Prescription Rationale

Chinese medical treatment for constipation is aimed at aiding digestion, eliminating excess Heat, and regulating the water content in the body.

Recommended Herbs

English Name	Pharmaceutical Name	Chinese Name
Microcos	Folium Microcos Paniculatae	*po bu ye*
Senna leaf	Folium Sennae	*fan xie ye*
Prunus seed	Semen Pruni	*yu li ren*
Betel nut	Semen Arecae Catechu	*bing lang*
Lonicera flower	Flos Lonicerae Japonicae	*jin yin hua*
Pueraria flower	Flos Puerariae	*ge hua*

Constipation, *continued*

Prevention

Maintain a balanced diet with enough fiber and water content
Consume more fruits and vegetables
Avoid overindulging in peppery, deep-fried, and barbecued foods
Avoid sitting for long periods, exercise daily
Maintain a regular daily schedule for emptying the bowels

Diabetes

Diabetes is a disorder in which the pancreas produces insufficient or no insulin. The symptoms include thirst, fatigue, weight loss, and high sugar content in the blood.

Prescription Rationale

In Chinese medicine, the treatment for diabetes emphasizes nourishing the spleen and the kidneys, reducing blood sugar, and regulating the water content of the body. There are no specific herbs known to directly address insulin deficiency. It is probable that the herbs work by indirectly stimulating insulin production.

Recommended Herbs

English Name	Pharmaceutical Name	Chinese Name
Peony	Radix Paeoniae Lactiflorae	*bai shao*
Chinese yam	Rhizoma Dioscoreae Oppositae	*shan yao*
Alpinia	Fructus Alpiniae Oxyphyllae	*yi zhi ren*
Corn silk	Stylus Zeae Mays	*yu mi xu*
Raw rehmannia	Radix Rehmanniae Glutinosae	*sheng di huang*
Astragalus	Radix Astragali Membranacei	*huang qi*
Plantago	Herba Plantaginis	*che qian cao*
Akebia	Caulis Mutong	*mu tong*
Polygonatum	Rhizoma Polygonati Odorati	*yu zhu*
Coptis	Rhizoma Coptidis	*huang lian*
Scrophularia	Radix Scrophulariae Ningpoensis	*xuan shen*

Diarrhea

Diarrhea is the frequent discharge of watery stools. If the diarrhea is not stopped, dehydration and progressive weakening of the body may ensue. Diarrhea can be caused by contaminated or spoiled food, coarse or highly seasoned food, or by overindulgence of alcohol for some individuals.

Prescription Rationale

Herbal treatment of diarrhea consists of clearing the digestive system of unwanted food, and reinvigorating the digestive system.

Recommended Herbs

English Name	Pharmaceutical Name	Chinese Name
Hawthorn fruit	Fructus Crataegi	*shan zha*
Ash bark	Cortex Fraxini	*qin pi*
Atractylodes	Rhizoma Atractylodis Macrocephalae	*bai zhu*
Peony	Radix Paeoniae Lactiflorae	*bai shao*
Rice sprout	Fructus Oryzae Sativae Germinatus	*gu ya*
Saussurea	Radix Aucklandiae Lappae	*mu xiang*
Chinaberry	Fructus Meliae Toosendan	*chuan lian zi*
Chicken gizzard internal lining	Endothelium Corneum Gigeriae Galli	*ji nei jin*
Licorice	Radix Glycyrrhizae Uralensis	*gan cao*

Prevention

Ensure food is clean and unspoiled before consumption
Avoid excessive alcohol consumption

Energy Enhancement

Low energy can be manifested by fatigue, apathy, difficulty in concentration, drowsiness, and feeling low-spirited.

Prescription Rationale

Lack of energy is a common phenomenon when the Yin and Yang of the body are not in balance. This means that the organs are not functioning harmoniously. Blood circulation is not at its best. Consequently, the flow of Qi throughout the body is slowed. The herbs in the following formula are aimed at restoring the organs to their normal functions.

Recommended Herbs

English Name	Pharmaceutical Name	Chinese Name
Peony	Radix Paeoniae Lactiflorae	*bai shao*
Tang-kuei	Radix Angelicae Sinensis	*dang gui*
Raw rehmannia	Radix Rehmanniae Glutinosae	*sheng di huang*
Codonopsis	Radix Codonopsitis Pilosulae	*dang shen*
Cistanche	Herba Cistanchis Deserticolae	*rou cong rong*
Antler glue sediment	Cornu Cervi Degelatinatium	*lu jiao shuang*
Cornus	Fructus Corni Officinalis	*shan zhu yu*
Psoralea	Fructus Psoraleae Corylifoliae	*bu gu zhi*
Alisma	Rhizoma Alismatis Orientalis	*ze xie*
Mulberry	Fructus Mori Albae	*sang shen*
Atractylodes	Rhizoma Atractylodis Macrocephalae	*bai zhu*
Chinese yam	Rhizoma Dioscoreae Oppositae	*shan yao*
Poria	Sclerotium Poriae Cocos	*fu ling*
Licorice	Radix Glycyrrhizae Uralensis	*gan cao*

Fertility Enhancement For Men

Male infertility can be caused by various factors such as low sperm count, impotence, among others.

Prescription Rationale

Chinese medical treatment emphasizes restoring the body to its normal balanced condition. According to Chinese medicine, infertility in men is the result of deficiency of vital energy in the kidneys, various deficiencies in the blood, and a weak reproductive organ.

Recommended Herbs

English Name	Pharmaceutical Name	Chinese Name
Rehmannia	Radix Rehmanniae Glutinosae Conquitae	*shu di huang*
Kirin ginseng	Radix Ginseng	*ji lin shen*
Tang-kuei	Radix Angelicae Sinensis	*dang gui*
Astragalus	Radix Astragali Membranacei	*huang qi*
Cinnamon bark	Cortex Cinnamomi Cassiae	*rou gui*
Cardamon	Fructus Amomi	*sha ren*
Psoralea	Fructus Psoraleae Corylifoliae	*bu gu zhi*
Morinda	Radix Morindae Officinalis	*ba ji tian*
Eucommia	Cortex Eucommiae Ulmoidis	*du zhong*
Cistanche	Herba Cistanchis Deserticolae	*rou cong rong*
Cynomorium	Herba Cynomorii Songarici	*suo yang*
Antler glue sediment	Cornu Cervi Degelatinatium	*lu jiao shuang*

Fertility Enhancement For Women

As in the male counterpart, female infertility is also due to a variety of factors resulting from the loss of balance in body functions.

Prescription Rationale

Chinese medical treatment of female infertility is aimed at restoring the body to its normal balanced condition. According to Chinese medicine, infertility in women is often due to insufficient vital energy in the kidneys, various deficiencies in the blood, and weak reproductive organs.

Recommended Herbs

English Name	Pharmaceutical Name	Chinese Name
Tang-kuei	Radix Angelicae Sinensis	dang gui
Chinese raspberry	Fructus Rubi Chingii	fu pen zi
Antler glue sediment	Cornu Cervi Degelatinatium	lu jiao shuang
Rehmannia	Radix Rehmanniae Glutinosae Conquitae	shu di huang
Kirin ginseng	Radix Ginseng	ji lin shen
Evodia	Fructus Evodiae Rutaecarpae	wu zhu yu
Zanthoxylum	Pericarpium Zanthoxyli Bungeani	chuan jiao
Poria spirit	Sclerotium Poriae Cocos Pararadicis	fu shen
Epimedium	Herba Epimedii	xian ling pi
Ligusticum	Radix Ligustici Chuanxiong	chuan xiong
Eucommia	Cortex Eucommiae Ulmoidis	du zhong
Morinda	Radix Morindae Officinalis	ba ji tian
Ligustrum	Fructus Ligustri Lucidi	nu zhen zi
Cynomorium	Herba Cynomorii Songarici	suo yang

Fibroid

Fibroid is a benign tumor that occurs in the walls of the uterus, and is made up of connective tissue and smooth muscle bundles.

Prescription Rationale

In Chinese medicine, fibroids are considered to be caused by blood stasis. Treatment involves reinvigorating the blood circulation, removing blood stagnancy, and promoting the vital energy of the body.

Recommended Herbs

English Name	Pharmaceutical Name	Chinese Name
Tang-kuei	Radix Angelica Sinensis	*dang gui*
Anteater scales	Squama Manitis Pentadactylae	*chuan shan jia*
Peach seed	Semen Persicae	*tao ren*
Raw rehmannia	Radix Rehmanniae Glutinosae	*sheng di huang*
Notoginseng	Radix Notoginseng	*san qi*
Moutan	Cortex Moutan Radicis	*mu dan pi*
Isatis root	Radix Isatidis seu Baphicacanthi	*ban lan gen*
Ligustrum	Fructus Ligustri Lucidi	*nu zhen zi*
Ligusticum	Radix Ligustici Chuanxiong	*chuan xiong*
Red Peony	Radix Paeoniae Rubrae	*chi shao*
Cinnamon twig	Ramulus Cinnamomi Cassiae	*gui zhi*
Cyperus	Rhizoma Cyperi Rotundi	*xiang fu*
Clematis	Radix Clematidis	*wei ling xian*
Lycopium	Herba Lycopi Lucidi	*ze lan*

Hemorrhoids

Hemorrhoids are distended veins in the lining of the anus. A variety of causes lead to the development of hemorrhoids, including pregnancy, constipation, straining during bowel movements, anal infection, excess Heat and Dampness in the body. Inflamed hemorrhoidal tissues usually result in pain, itching and bleeding.

Prescription Rationale

Hemorrhoids can be controlled by Chinese herbs although a complete cure requires longterm treatment. Treatment strategy consists of nourishing and cleansing the blood, alleviating Heat and Dampness in the body, reducing inflammation of the hemorrhoidal tissues, and stopping the bleeding.

Recommended Herbs

English Name	Pharmaceutical Name	Chinese Name
Peony	Radix Paeoniae Lactiflorae	*bai shao*
Tang-kuei	Radix Angelicae Sinensis	*dang gui*
Raw rehmannia	Radix Rehmanniae Glutinosae	*sheng di huang*
Fraxinus	Cortex Fraxini	*qin pi*
Phellodendron	Cortex Phellodendri	*huang bai*
Lonicera flower	Flos Lonicerae Japonicae	*jin yin hua*
Sophora flower	Flos Sophorae Japonicae Immaturus	*huai hua*
Drosera	Herba Droserae Burmanni	*jin di luo*
Sanguisorba	Radix Sanguisorbae officinalis	*di yu*
Pulsatilla	Radix Pulsatillae Chinensis	*bai tou weng*

Hemorrhoids, *continued*

Prevention

Practise good hygiene to prevent tissue infection

Avoid or moderate intake of peppery, deep-fried, and barbecued foods in order to reduce heat in the body

Follow a balanced diet that includes plenty of fruits and vegetables to prevent irregularity

Avoid seafood such as crab and certain shellfish which may cause build-up of Dampness and Heat in the body

High Blood Pressure

Hypertension is abnormally high blood pressure and may be due to obesity, stress, older age, excess alcohol intake, and various disorders of the kidney, among others. Western medical treatment usually produces side effects such as dizziness, palpitation, and fatigue. Furthermore, patients often develop a dependency on the prescribed drugs.

Prescription Rationale

Chinese medical theory considers high blood pressure as the presence of excess Heat in the liver and the blood. The Heat rises and causes hyperactivity of the heart. The herbs in the formula below are used to reduce Heat and calm the heart. These herbs produce few side effects. When the patient's condition improves, the prescription can be terminated.

Recommended Herbs

English Name	Pharmaceutical Name	Chinese Name
Raw rehmannia	Radix Rehmanniae Glutinosae	*sheng di huang*
Gastrodia	Rhizoma Gastrodiae Elatae	*tian ma*
Motherwort	Herba Leonuri Heterophylli	*yi mu cao*
Achyranthes	Radix Achyranthis Bidentatae	*niu xi*
Eucommia	Cortex Eucommiae Ulmoidis	*du zhong*
Gentian	Radix Gentianae Longdancao	*long dan cao*
Loranthus	Ramulus Sangjisheng	*sang ji sheng*
Siler	Radix Ledebouriellae Divaricatae	*fang feng*
Uncaria	Ramulus Uncariae cum Uncis	*gou teng*
Fleeceflower root	Radix Polygoni Multiflori	*he shou wu*
Poria spirit	Sclerotium Poriae Cocos Pararadicis	*fu shen*

High Blood Pressure, *continued*

Prevention

Maintain a balanced diet
Avoid foods with high fat or cholesterol content
Avoid stress
Exercise regularly
Maintain a balance between work and relaxation

Influenza

Influenza (or flu) has the following symptoms: fever, headache, joint pain, coughing, nasal congestion, phlegm, fatigue, feeling of alternating heat and chills, among others.

Prescription Rationale

Traditional Chinese treatment for influenza consists of relieving the symptoms such as fever and cough. In addition, herbs are used to regulate water metabolism and strengthen the body so that it is able to combat the illness.

Recommended Herbs

English Name	Pharmaceutical Name	Chinese Name
Ephedra	Herba Ephedrae	*ma huang*
Gypsum	Gypsum	*shi gao*
Eupatorium	Herba Eupatorii Haplocalycis	*pei lan*
Forsythia fruit	Fructus Forsythiae Suspensae	*lian qiao*
Apricot seed	Semen Armeniacae Pruni	*xing ren*
Fritillaria	Bulbus Fritillariae Thunbergii	*zhe bei mu*
Peucedanum	Radix Peucedani	*qian hu*
Ginger skin	Cortex Zingiberis Officinalis Recens	*jiang pi*
Scrophularia	Radix Scrophulariae Ningpoensis	*xuan shen*
Licorice	Radix Glycyrrhizae Uralensis	*gan cao*

Prevention

Protect the body against hot and cold weather
Get plenty of rest

Insomnia

Insomnia can be any one or a combination of the following: taking a long time to fall asleep, easy awakening during sleep, dream-disturbed sleep, and not feeling rested after a night's sleep. Common causes of insomina are anxiety, stress in the work place, worry about a problem, or fear about the occurrence of something undesirable.

Prescription Rationale

Herbal treatment involves sedating the body, nourishing the blood and clearing excess Heat, balancing the body functions, and stimulating the appetite.

Recommended Herbs

English Name	Pharmaceutical Name	Chinese Name
Biota seed	Semen Biotae Orientalis	*bai zi ren*
Albizzia	Cortex Albizziae Julibrissin	*he huan pi*
Polygala	Radix Polygalae Tenuifoliae	*yuan zhi*
Dragon bone	Os Draconis	*long gu*
Salvia	Radix Salviae Miltiorrhizae	*dan shen*
Poria	Sclerotium Poriae Cocos	*fu ling*
Tang-kuei	Radix Angelicae Sinensis	*dang gui*
Gelatin	Gelatinum Corii Asini	*e jiao*
Peony	Radix Paeoniae Lactiflorae	*bai shao*
Raw rehmannia	Radix Rehmanniae Glutinosae	*sheng di huang*
Codonopsis	Radix Codonopsitis Pilosulae	*dang shen*
Astragalus	Radix Astragali Membranacei	*huang qi*
Light wheat	Semen Tritici Aestivi Levis	*fu xiao mai*
Anemarrhena	Rhizoma Anemarrhenae Asphodeloidis	*zhi mu*
Atractylodes	Rhizoma Atractylodis Macrocephalae	*bai zhu*
Licorice	Radix Glycyrrhizae Uralensis	*gan cao*

Insomnia, *continued*

Prevention

Avoid stress and learn relaxation techniques
Enjoy the simple things of life such as eating, exercise, and hobbies
Maintain a regular schedule of work and relaxation
Maintain a balanced diet

Longevity

Chinese folklore is full of stories about the quest for longevity. Some herbs are thought to produce longevity but their effects are difficult to prove. On the other hand, many herbs are quite effective for the maintenance of good health during old age if taken on a regular basis. What is important is not how long one wants to live, but how much happiness or satisfaction one can derive from life. To be able to fully enjoy life, one needs to have good health. The following formula enables persons over age 50 to overcome general physical weakness, and to carry on activities they formerly participated in.

Prescription Rationale

As an individual ages, the vital parts of the body gradually weaken, blood circulation slows, and the entire system is inclined toward disharmony. A delicate balance of herbs taken regularly can help a person regain vitality and delay the occurrence of the physical conditions due to old age.

Prescription Rationale

English Name	Pharmaceutical Name	Chinese Name
Tang-kuei	Radix Angelicae Sinensis	*dang gui*
Fleeceflower root	Radix Polygoni Multiflori	*he shou wu*
Chinese raspberry	Fructus Rubi Chingii	*fu pen zi*
Kirin ginseng	Radix Ginseng	*ji lin shen*
Rehmannia	Radix Rehmanniae Glutinosae Conquitae	*shu di huang*
Lycium fruit	Fructus Lycii	*gou qi zi*
Eucommia	Cortex Eucommiae Ulmoidis	*du zhong*
Antler glue sediment	Cornu Cervi Degelatinatium	*lu jiao shuang*
Euryale	Semen Euryales Ferocis	*qian shi*

Longevity, *continued*

English Name	Pharmaceutical Name	Chinese Name
Morinda	Radix Morindae Officinalis	*ba ji tian*
Rose fruit	Fructus Rosae Laevigatae	*jin ying zi*
Cuscuta	Semen Cuscutae Chinensis	*tu si zi*
Psoralea	Fructus Psoraleae Corylifoliae	*bu gu zhi*
Cornus	Fructus Corni Officinalis	*shan zhu yu*
Lotus seed	Semen Nelumbinis Nuciferae	*lian zi*
Fennel	Fructus Foeniculi Vulgaris	*xiao hui xiang*
Ganoderma	Ganoderma Lucidum	*ling zhi*

Menopause

Menopause is the cessation of menstruation which occurs in women between the ages of 45 and 55. This is a natural process as a result of reduced production of estrogen hormones by the ovaries. A woman going through menopause is subject to various kinds of physical and emotional stresses.

Prescription Rationale

Menopause is not an illness but a natural physical phenomenon. Treatment is aimed at helping the woman overcome the physical and emotional stresses through a delicate balance of herbs that nourish the blood, regulate the body fluids, relieve stress and anxiety, and strengthen the liver and kidneys.

Recommended Herbs

English Name	Pharmaceutical Name	Chinese Name
Tang-kuei	Radix Angelicae Sinensis	*dang gui*
Curcuma root	Tuber Curcumae	*yu jin*
Fleeceflower root	Radix Polygoni Multiflori	*he shou wu*
American ginseng	Radix Panacis Quinguefolii	*xi yang shen*
Rhubarb	Radix et Rhizoma Rhei	*da huang*
Biota seed	Semen Biotae Orientalis	*bai zi ren*
Polygala	Radix Polygalae Tenuifoliae	*yuan zhi*
Poria spirit	Sclerotium Poriae Cocos Pararadicis	*fu shen*
Swallowwort	Radix Cynanchi Baiwei	*bai wei*
Wolfberry bark	Cortex Lycii Radicis	*di gu pi*
Gentian	Radix Gentianae Longdancao	*long dan cao*
Peony	Radix Paeoniae Lactiflorae	*bai shao*
Raw rehmannia	Radix Rehmanniae Glutinosae	*sheng di huang*
Cornus	Fructus Corni Officinalis	*shan zhu yu*

Menstrual Discomfort

The common problems during menstruation are pain, muscle tension, excessive bleeding, anxiety, and fatigue. Irregular menstruation is also a source of stress for many women.

Prescription Rationale

To relieve menstrual discomfort, the herbs in the following formula are used to stop the pain, regulate the menstrual flow, and relax the muscles. The herbs can also nourish the blood after menstruation ends.

Recommended Herbs

English Name	Pharmaceutical Name	Chinese Name
Raw rehmannia	Radix Rehmanniae Glutinosae	*sheng di huang*
Tang-kuei	Radix Angelicae Sinensis	*dang gui*
Moutan	Cortex Moutan Radicis	*mu dan pi*
Red peony	Radix Paeoniae Rubrae	*chi shao*
Lycopium	Herba Lycopi Lucidi	*ze lan*
Ligusticum	Radix Ligustici Chuanxiong	*chuan xiong*
Nutgrass	Rhizoma Cyperi Rotundi	*xiang fu*
Motherwort	Herba Leonuri Heterophylli	*yi mu cao*
Frankincense	Gummi Olibanum	*ru xiang*
Myrrh	Myrrha	*mo yao*
Scutellaria	Radix Scutellariae Baicalensis	*huang qin*
Dipacus	Radix Dipsaci Asperi	*xu duan*

Migraine

Migraine is a severe headache often, but not always, located at one or both temples, often accompanied by nausea and vomiting. Preceding the headache, transient symptoms occur, which include loss of vision, defective speech or body movements, and illusions of flashing lights. There is no single cause, although there appears to be a familial tendency.

Prescription Rationale

Chinese medical theory attributes the cause of headache to the harmful factor of Wind affecting the head and harbored within the blood. Herbal treatment involves dispelling the Wind and nourishing the blood. In addition, herbs are used to calm the nerves and consolidate the vital energy of the body.

Recommended Herbs

English Name	Pharmaceutical Name	Chinese Name
Tang-kuei	Radix Angelicae Sinensis	dang gui
Ligusticum	Radix Ligustici Chuanxiong	chuan xiong
Hornet nest	Nidus Vespae	lu feng fang
Dahurica	Radix Angelicae Dahuricae	bai zhi
Fresh ginger	Rhizoma Zingiberis Officinalis Recens	sheng jiang
Notopterygium	Rhizoma et Radix Notopterygii	qiang huo
Astragalus	Radix Astragali Membranacei	huang qi
Poria spirit	Sclerotium Poriae Cocos Pararadicis	fu shen
Codonopsis	Radix Codonopsitis Pilosulae	dang shen
Licorice	Radix Glycyrrhizae Uralensis	gan cao

Skin Irritations

Skin irritations are usually signs of developing skin ailments. If left untreated or not treated properly, the irritation can spread and/or develop into a more serious condition. Irritations are characterized by itching, swelling, dryness of the skin, as well as other symptoms. Scratching of the affected area only worsens the conditions.

Prescription Rationale

Skin irritations usually result from a changed nature of the blood which then affects the skin. The herbs in the following formula are used to cleanse the blood, strengthen the liver, reduce itching, and nourish the skin.

Recommended Herbs

English Name	Pharmaceutical Name	Chinese Name
Lonicera flower	Flos Lonicerae Japonicae	jin yin hua
Pueraria	Radix Puerariae Japonicae	ge gen
Scutellaria	Radix Scutellariae Baicalensis	huang qin
Viola	Herba cum Radice Violae Yedoensitis	zi hua di ding
Gentian	Radix Gentianae Longdancao	long dan cao
Smilax	Rhizoma Smilacis Glabrae	tu fu ling
Peony	Radix Paeoniae Lactiflorae	bai shao
Curcuma	Tuber Curcumae	yu jin
Abrus	Herba Abri Fruticulosis	ji gu cao

Prevention

Keep the skin clean
Avoid spicy foods and alcohol
Be aware of which foods cause skin hypersensitivity

Stress Relief

Everyone is subject to the stresses of daily life to a certain degree. The human body is able to handle various kinds of stress, but in some cases, the stress may reach an unbearable level that forces an individual to seek medical help.

Prescription Rationale

Because of their broad effects on the body, Chinese herbs are effective for stress relief. The herbs in the formula below help to calm the nerves, relax the muscles, balance the functions of the vital organs, regulate the blood flow, and consolidate the vital energy of the body.

Recommended Herbs

English Name	Pharmaceutical Name	Chinese Name
Tang-kuei	Radix Angelicae Sinensis	*dang gui*
Peony root bark	Cortex Moutan Radicis	*mu dan pi*
Polygala	Radix Polygalae Tenuifoliae	*yuan zhi*
Atractylodes	Rhizoma Atractylodis Macrocephalae	*bai zhu*
Biota seed	Semen Biotae Orientalis	*bai zi ren*
Ganoderma	Ganoderma Lucidum	*ling zhi*
Dragon bone	Os Draconis	*long gu*
Astragalus	Radix Astragali Membranacei	*huang qi*
Gardenia fruit	Fructus Gardeniae Jasminoidis	*zhi zi*
Peony	Radix Paeoniae Lactiflorae	*bai shao*
Raw rehmannia	Radix Rehmanniae Glutinosae	*sheng di huang*

Weight Control

How a person views his/her body weight is a subjective matter. But, from a health viewpoint, when body weight becomes excessive, it may cause heart problems and other related ailments.

Prescription Rationale

Body weight depends on the amount of food essence (including fat) that remains in the body. In general, increasing the metabolism of the body will lower the weight. Weight control can be done by using herbs to stimulate the digestive system, and invigorate the vital energy of the body.

Recommended Herbs

English Name	Pharmaceutical Name	Chinese Name
Betel nut	Semen Arecae Catechu	*bing lang*
Magnolia bark	Cortex Magnoliae Officinalis	*hou po*
Rhubarb	Radix et Rhizoma Rhei	*da huang*
Areca peel	Pericarpium Arecae Catechu	*da fu pi*
Microcos	Folium Microcos Paniculatae	*po bu ye*
Star anise	Fructus Illicii	*ba jiao hui xiang*
Saussurea	Radix Aucklandiae Lappae	*mu xiang*
Chinaberry	Fructus Meliae Toosendan	*chuan lian zi*
Shield fern	Rhizoma Guanzhong	*guan zhong*

Prevention

Maintain a balanced diet; do not overeat
Maintain a regular exercise schedule
Engage in more outdoor activities

Yin-Type Weakness

Yin-type weakness is a physical discomfort mainly due to change of weather to a cooler and damper climate. When a person ages, such discomforts may worsen.

Prescription Rationale

Yin-type weakness is a result of an imbalance between the body and the external environment. In this case, Yin is dominant both inside and outside the body. Chinese herbs that promote the Yang can be used to help restore the body to equilibrium. The following prescription is a general "tune up" formula to improve blood circulation, raise the energy level, and dispel the chill and dampness within the body. The prescription can be taken regularly especially during the cold or rainy season.

Recommended Herbs

English Name	Pharmaceutical Name	Chinese Name
Kirin ginseng	Radix Ginseng	*ji lin shen*
Schisandra	Fructus Schisandrae Chinensis	*wu wei zi*
Tang-kuei	Radix Angelicae Sinensis	*dang gui*
Polygala	Radix Polygalae Tenuifoliae	*yuan zhi*
Ophiopogon	Radix Ophiopogonis Japonici	*mai men dong*
Raw rehmannia	Radix Rehmanniae Glutinosae	*sheng di huang*
Anemarrhena	Rhizoma Anemarrhenae Asphodeloidis	*zhi mu*
Poria	Sclerotium Poriae Cocos	*fu ling*
Atractylodes	Rhizoma Atractylodis Macrocephalae	*bai zhu*
Licorice	Radix Glycyrrhizae Uralensis	*gan cao*

Yin-Type Weakness, *continued*

Prevention

Avoid or decrease intake of ice-cold foods
Lead a more active life

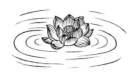

Chapter 8

Prevention And Self-Help

The Wisdom Of Prevention

Prevention as a survival method is as old as the human race. Advances in medical science tend to eclipse the importance of prevention; but such advances can never take the place of prevention as a cost-effective means of health care, for prevention has a great deal to do with lifestyle rather than medicine. Thus, we must not neglect the value of prevention especially in this era of increasing medical costs. Practicing prevention is just a way of self-help toward achieving a healthier and happier life.

Prevention requires the realization that humans are but part of nature, and are not created just to perform certain functions like a machine. We are here to enrich all other living and non-living things of nature, as they do for us. Hence, to live in harmony with nature is what the life process is all about. We can easily see the extensive damage to our health when we pollute the environment. We are the ones to suffer when we disrupt the balance of nature.

Prevention means that there must be a balance between work, eating, relaxation, exercise, and rest. Moderation is the key for achieving a balance, because moderation prevents excesses. Practicing prevention raises our consciousness about our physical and emotional conditions, and helps us understand more about our external environment such as the weather, changes of which can affect our health. Through prevention, we can learn more about the relationships between ourselves and the things that surround us. Prevention requires a conscious effort and discipline, but the payoff will be great in terms of good health and happiness.

Over the past decades, Western medical technology has enabled the administration of collective prevention for the masses. Vaccines against smallpox and measles have contributed significantly to prevention. But vaccines can only prevent a limited number of diseases. Furthermore, with Western medicine, more resources are directed toward treatment than toward prevention, and the benefits to the consumer are restricted because of the high cost of medical services.

In Chinese medicine, prevention has always been equally important as treatment, or even more important. Various methods of prevention have been developed and refined through the centuries, and their wide acceptance has made them part of Chinese culture and folklore. Many Westerners are already familiar with Tai Chi and Qi Gong. Apart from physical exercise, many Chinese herbs have preventive effects. Because such herbs are inexpensive, they can be used on a daily basis. When used in moderation, the herbs are gentle and mild, so that side effects are non-existent. Another advantage of herbs is that they do not create dependency, and can be discontinued any time after they have achieved the intended effects. Finally, many herbs can be incorporated as ingredients into daily cooking to enhance the taste, nutrition, and medicinal value of foods.

In the remainder of this chapter, some Chinese health foods like soup, rice porridge, and sweet soup are introduced. Such foods constitute an important part of the Chinese diet. Besides their nutritional and medicinal values, they are inexpensive and easy to prepare.

The Goodness Of Soup

Soup is nutritious and easy to make. Just gather the ingredients, combine them in the right proportions, and boil them in water. The relative quantities of water and ingredients will determine the thickness of the soup. Westerners seem to prefer thick soups, whereas Chinese prefer to drink the broth and consume the ingredients separately.

Soup normally comes before the principal dish in a Western meal. In the Chinese tradition, especially in the south, soup stands on its own. It can be served at mealtimes with a meal, in between meals, or as a snack before bedtime. Since soup is an important part of the diet, the Chinese have developed a wide range of soup recipes. The Cantonese in particular are well known for their enthusiasm for soup, and for the great variety of their soup menus.

With the addition of some special herbs, soup can be eaten in order to prevent ailments or address certain physical conditions. The soups described below are selected recipes used by our family through the years. Most of the ingredients can be purchased from Asian supermarkets, and the special herbs from any herb store. When the soup is done, the essence of the ingredients will have been dissolved in the broth. Therefore, the broth should be consumed. The boiled ingredients may be eaten as well, with the exception of some herbs which will be rendered coarse and tasteless after cooking. Specific instructions in each of the following recipes describe which herbs to discard.

General weakness.

This soup may be eaten to promote energy, appetite, and concentration; the following recipe is suitable for children and the elderly, too.

Ingredients:

½	chicken, without skin, separate the wing, leg and breast (8 oz. lean beef, ground or sliced, may be substituted for chicken)
4 oz	longan fruit, dried (Arillus Euphoria Longanae, *long yan rou*)
4 oz	Chinese yam, dried (Radix Dioscoreae Oppositae, *shan yao*)
4 oz	lycium fruit, dried (Fructus Lycii, *gou qi zi*)
3 cups	water

After the soup boils, let it simmer for 3 to 4 hours. Add boiling water to compensate for evaporation. Skim the fat floating on top of the broth. Salt or soy sauce may be added to enhance the taste. Drink the broth, and consume all the other ingredients.

Nourishment and strength.

This soup may be eaten to expedite recovery after an illness, surgery, or chemotherapy.

Ingredients:

½	chicken, without skin, separate the wing, leg and breast
4 oz	fish stomach
6 oz	sea cucumber, sliced
4 oz	caterpillar fungus (Cordyceps Sinensis, *dong chong xia cao*)
3 cups	water

After the soup boils, let it simmer for 3 to 4 hours. Add boiling water to compensate for evaporation. Skim the fat floating on top of the broth. Salt or soy sauce may be added to enhance the taste. Drink the broth, and consume all the other ingredients.

Ache and pain of the joints.

This soup may be eaten to prevent fatigue, over-exertion, and the onset of arthritis.

Ingredients:

1	whole or ½ carp
5 oz	coix seed (Semen Coicis Lachryma-jobi, *yi yi ren*)
4 oz	mulberry branch (Ramulus Mori Alba, *sang zhi*)
4 oz	pueraria root (Radix Puerariae, *ge gen*)
3 cups	water

After the soup boils, let it simmer for 1 to 2 hours. Add boiling water to compensate for evaporation. Salt or soy sauce may be added to enhance the taste. Drink the broth, and consume the fish and the coix seed.

Blood nourishment.

This soup may be eaten to prevent anemia, and to replenish milk for lactating women.

Ingredients:

1	whole or ½ catfish
5 oz	black beans, dried
3 cups	water

After the soup boils, let it simmer for 1 to 2 hours. Add boiling water to compensate for evaporation. Salt or soy sauce may be added to enhance the taste. Drink the broth, and consume all the other ingredients.

Strengthen the heart and lungs.

This soup may be eaten to prevent aging weakness in adults and
the elderly.

Ingredients:

1	whole pigeon, separate the legs, wings, and breast
5 oz	American ginseng, sliced (Radix Panacis Quinquefolii, *xi yang shen*)
3 cups	water

After the soup boils, let it simmer for 2 to 3 hours. Add boiling
water to compensate for evaporation. Skim the fat floating on top
of the broth. Salt or soy sauce may be added to enhance the taste.
Drink the broth, and consume all the other ingredients.

Strengthen the liver.

Ingredients:

3 oz	pig liver, sliced
7 oz	lean pork, sliced
5 oz	abrus (Herba Abri Fruticulosis, *ji gu cao*)
3 cups	water

After the soup boils, let it simmer for 2 to 3 hours. Add boiling
water to compensate for evaporation. Skim the fat floating on top
of the broth. Salt or soy sauce may be added to enhance the taste.
Drink the broth, and consume all the other ingredients except the
herb.

Strengthen the kidneys and lungs.

Ingredients:

½	duck, without skin, separate the wing, leg, and breast
5 oz	caterpillar fungus (Cordyceps Sinensis, *dong chong xia cao*)
3 cups	water

After the soup boils, let it simmer for 2 to 3 hours. Add boiling water to compensate for evaporation. Skim the fat floating on top of the broth. Salt or soy sauce may be added to enhance the taste. Drink the broth, and consume all the other ingredients.

Strengthen the lungs and the respiratory tract.

This soup may be eaten to prevent and relieve coughing, phlegm, and asthma.

Ingredients:

7 oz	lean pork, sliced
8 pieces	figs, dried, cut into halves
4 oz	almond, south type (Semen Pruni Armeniacae, *tian xing ren*)
4 oz	almond, north type (Semen Pruni Armeniacae, *ku xing ren*)
2	momordica fruits, cut into halves (Fructus Momordicae Grosvenori, *luo han guo*)
3 cups	water

After the soup boils, let it simmer for 2 to 3 hours. Add boiling water to compensate for evaporation. Skim the fat floating on top of the broth. Salt or soy sauce may be added to enhance the taste. Drink the broth, and consume all the other ingredients except the almonds and momordica fruit.

Excess heat in the body.

This soup may be eaten to prevent and relieve fever and other flu symptoms.

Ingredients:

8 oz	bok choi, sliced
8 oz	carrots, sliced
10 pieces	water chestnut, cut into halves
5 pieces	figs, dried, cut into halves
3 cups	water

After the soup boils, let it simmer for 2 to 3 hours. Add boiling water to compensate for evaporation. Salt or soy sauce may be added to enhance the taste. Drink the broth, and consume all the other ingredients.

Yin-type weakness.

This soup may be eaten to prevent colds, anemia, lack of energy and appetite, and is most suitable for the elderly.

Ingredients:

8 oz	lamb, sliced (8 oz lean beef, sliced, may be substituted)
3 oz	ginger, sliced
10 pieces	red dates
5 oz	sugar cane, available in can
4 oz	Tang-kuei (Radix Angelica Sinensis, *dang gui*)
4 oz	astragalus (Radix Astragali Membranacei, *huang qi*)
3 cups	water

After the soup boils, let it simmer for 2 to 3 hours. Add boiling water to compensate for evaporation. Skim the fat floating on top of the broth. Salt or soy sauce may be added to enhance the taste. Drink the broth, and consume the meat and the dates only.

Anxiety and nervousness.

This soup may be eaten to calm the body and mind, and prevent insomnia.

Ingredients:
     6 oz   lean pork, sliced
15 pieces   red dates
     3 cups   water

After the soup boils, let it simmer for 2 to 3 hours. Add boiling water to compensate for evaporation. Skim the fat floating on top of the broth. Salt or soy sauce may be added to enhance the taste. Drink the broth, and consume all the other ingredients.

Indigestion and lack of appetite.

This soup may be eaten to promote digestion and restore the appetite.

Ingredients:
     6 oz   pig stomach, sliced
     4 oz   octopus, dried
     3 oz   black pepper grains
     3 cups   water

After the soup boils, let it simmer for 3 to 4 hours. Add boiling water to compensate for evaporation. Skim the fat floating on top of the broth. Salt or soy sauce may be added to enhance the taste. Drink the broth, and consume all other ingredients except the pepper.

Irregular menstruation or hemorrhoid bleeding.

This soup may be eaten to regulate blood flow and prevent the loss of blood.

Ingredients:

10 pieces	red dates
5 oz	Black Tremella mushroom *(mu er)*
5 oz	Tang-kuei (Radix Angelicae Sinensis, *dang gui*)
3 cups	water

After the soup boils, let it simmer for 3 to 4 hours. Add boiling water to compensate for evaporation. Salt or soy sauce may be added to enhance the taste. Drink the broth, and consume all other ingredients except the herb.

Health maintenance.

This soup may be eaten to replenish vigor and energy.

Ingredients:

½	chicken, without skin, separate the leg, wings and breast
4 oz	abalone, sliced
4 oz	Korean ginseng (Radix Ginseng, *gao li shen*)
4 oz	achyranthes (Radix Achyranthis Bidentatae, *niu xi*)
4 oz	eucommia (Cortex Eucommiae Ulmoidis, *du zhong*)
3 cups	water

After the soup boils, let it simmer for 3 to 4 hours. Add boiling water to compensate for evaporation. Skim the fat floating on top of the broth. Salt or soy sauce may be added to enhance the taste. Drink the broth, and consume all other ingredients except the herbs.

Postnatal care.

This soup may be eaten to recover after giving birth.

Ingredients:

½	chicken, without skin, separate the wing, leg, and breast
4 oz	ginger, sliced
5 oz	black mushroom
4 oz	Black Tremella mushroom *(mu er)*
3 oz	lilyflower, dried
3 cups	rice wine

This special soup is made with rice wine rather than water. After the soup boils, let it simmer for 2 to 3 hours. Add boiling water or rice wine to adjust the alcohol content of the soup. Skim the fat floating on top of the broth. Drink the broth. Salt may be added to enhance the taste. Consume all the other ingredients.

The Convenience Of Rice Porridge

Rice porridge is a popular meal in China, especially in the south. Porridge is soft and light, and consequently is easily digested. Individuals with poor digestions, who are overweight, or who are ill or convalescing, find porridge a soothing, light meal. For healthy people, rice porridge is a delightful meal suitable for breakfast, lunch or as a bedtime snack. It is nutritious but does not give one a heavy feeling after consumption, since it requires no oil nor fat in its preparation.

Porridge is made by simmering rice in water. To start out, add one cup of rice to three cups of water. When the water boils, lower the heat and allow the content to simmer for about an hour. Stir occasionally to prevent the rice from sticking to the bottom of the pot. The longer the simmering, the softer the porridge. The thickness of the porridge can be adjusted by adding water or allowing water to evaporate.

The resultant porridge is a base from which a great variety of light meals can be created by adding different combinations of meat and vegetables. This porridge base can be stored in the refrigerator for use during the next several days. To prepare for the porridge meal, slice the desired meat and vegetables, the raw meat may be marinated with soy sauce. Then spoon out a portion of the porridge base into a pot, and heat until boiling, stir occasionally. Add water if necessary to adjust the thickness of the porridge. When the porridge begins to boil, add the raw meat and vegetables and stir.

When the meat and vegetables are cooked, the porridge meal is ready. Salt or other seasoning may be added to enhance the taste. A small quantity of chopped scallions can also be added. If preferred, the meat and vegetables can be taken out of the porridge and eaten with soy sauce and sesame oil on the side.

The following are meat and vegetable combinations that are popular especially among the Cantonese. Any combination can be made by selecting one's favorite ingredients.

No-meat porridge.

Cleanses the digestive system after a heavy meal eaten the previous day, resulting in fullness or indigestion.

Ingredients:

1 serving	rice porridge base
4 oz	dried beancurd* stick (beancurd skin), cut into small pieces after soaking in water
7 pieces	ginko nuts, cut into halves

After boiling, simmer for 2 to 3 hours, add boiling water to adjust the thickness of the porridge. Salt may be added to enhance the taste.

*tofu skin (Fu Zhu)

Clear-heat porridge.

Combats heat discomforts such as persistent thirst, insomnia, and irritability.

Ingredients:

1 serving	rice porridge base
4 oz	lean pork, sliced
1	preserved egg (one-thousand-year egg), sliced into small pieces
3 oz	dried oyster

After boiling, simmer for 2 to 3 hours, add boiling water to adjust the thickness of the porridge. Salt may be added to enhance the taste.

Various combinations.

The following porridges are popular primarily for their good taste. They have no intended medicinal value.

Beef: sliced into thin pieces
Some sliced lettuce
1   raw egg, whipped

Cook in a boiling rice porridge base until the meat is done.

Pork: sliced into thin pieces (or use ground meat and form into small meat balls)
Liver and kidney, cut into thin slices
Some sliced lettuce

Cook in a boiling rice porridge base until the meat is done.

Chicken and abalone: Slice into thin pieces
Some sliced lettuce

Simmer for about an hour in a boiling rice porridge base.

Fish: Slice into thin pieces (any kind of fish will do)
Slices of beef may be added if desired
Some sliced lettuce

Cook in a boiling rice porridge base until the meat is done.

Other seafood: Prepare some shrimp, and some slices of fish or squid
Some sliced lettuce

Cook in a boiling rice porridge base until the seafood is done.

The Gentleness Of Sweet Soup

Sweet soup is a category of Chinese culinary delights largely unknown to the West. Some Chinese restaurants in America serve a sweet soup as dessert after a full dinner. However, sweet soup is more than only a dessert, for it can be a snack enjoyed any time during the day. Like rice porridge, sweet soup is more popular in southern China, especially in Canton.

Sweet soup is made in the same manner as ordinary soup except without meat. It is intended to promote health or relieve certain conditions, and has a gentle and long-term effect on the body, so it is suitable for consumption on a regular basis. As a snack before bedtime, sweet soup can help one sleep better while the digested ingredients slowly work their effects through the night.

Health maintenance.

Helps body adjust to sudden weather changes, and prevents conditions such as colds, cough, phlegm, persistent thirst, and the like.

Ingredients:

5 oz	coix seed (Semen Coicis Lachryma-jobi, *yi yi ren*)
4 oz	longan fruit, dried (Arillus Euphoriae Longanae, *long yan rou*)
4 oz	Chinese yam, dried (Rhizoma Dioscoreae oppositae, *shan yao*)
4 oz	polygonatum (Rhizoma Polygonati Odorati, *yu zhu*)
4 oz	euryale seed (Semen Euryales Feroces, *qian shi*)
4 oz	glehnia (Radix Adenophorae seu Glehniae, *sha shen*)
4 oz	lotus seed (Semen Nelumbinis Nuciferae, *lian zi*)
2	momordica fruits, cut into halves (Fructus Momordicae Grosvenori, *luo han guo*)
3 cups	water
	rock sugar, desired amount to suit taste

After the soup boils, simmer for 2 to 3 hours. Add boiling water if more broth is desired. Drink the broth. Consume the other ingredients with broth if desired.

Clear heat.

Relieves discomforts associated with excess heat in the body, including canker sores, constipation, hemorrhoid itching, sleeplessness, and the like.

Ingredients:

7 oz	green beans, dried
4 oz	kelp, sliced
3 oz	laminaria (Thallus Algae, *kun bu*)
3 cups	water
	rock sugar, desired amount to suit taste

After the soup boils, simmer for 3 to 4 hours. Add boiling water if more broth is desired. Consume all the ingredients. Add ice or refrigerate to make a cold snack if desired.

Nourishment.

Promotes health and nourishes the skin.

Ingredients:

4 oz	beancurd stick (beancurd skin), cut into small pieces after soaking in water
10	red dates, cut into halves
1	egg, whipped
4 oz	Chinese yam, dried (Radix Dioscoreae Oppositae, *shan yao*)
4 oz	polygonatum (Rhizoma Polygonati Odorati, *yu zhu*)
4 oz	lotus seed (Semen Nelumbinis Nuciferae, *lian zi*)
3 cups	water
	rock sugar, desired amount to suit taste

After the soup boils, simmer for 3 to 4 hours. Add boiling water if more broth is desired. Consume all the ingredients.

Strengthen the lungs and liver.

Relieves or prevents coughing.

Ingredients:
      8 oz   abrus (Herba Abri Fruticulosis, *ji gu cao*)
   3 cups   water
                brown sugar, desired amount to suit taste

After the soup boils, simmer for 1 to 2 hours. Add boiling water if more broth is desired. Drink the broth only.

Strengthen the digestive system.

Relieves indigestion and heat.

Ingredients:
10 pieces   water chestnut, cut into small pieces
      4 oz   beancurd stick (beancurd skin), cut into small pieces after
                soaking in water
   3 cups   water
                rock sugar, desired amount to suit taste

After the soup boils, simmer for 1 to 2 hours. Add boiling water if more broth is desired. Consume all the ingredients.

Promote sleep.

Ingredients:
      3 oz   White Tremella mushroom *(bai mu er)*
   2 cups   water
     1 cup   milk
                rock sugar, desired amount to suit taste

After the soup boils, simmer for 1 to 2 hours. Add the milk only when the soup is ready to be served. Consume all the ingredients.

Relieve coughing and phlegm.

Ingredients:
- 5 oz   almonds
- 4 oz   glehnia (Radix Adenophorae seu Glehniae, *sha shen*)
- 4 oz   polygonatum (Rhizoma Polygonati Odorati, *yu zhu*)
- 2   momordica fruits, cut into halves (Fructus Momordicae Grosvenori, *luo han guo*)
- 4 oz   pyrola (Herba Pyrolae, *lu xian cao*)
- 4 oz   fritillaria (Bulbus Fritillariae Cirrhosae, *chuan bei mu*)
- 3 cups   water
-    rock sugar, desired amount to suit taste

After the soup boils, simmer for 2 to 3 hours. Add boiling water if more broth is desired. Drink the broth only.

Regulate water metabolism.

Relieves discomfort due to dampness, also relieves urinary difficulty.

Ingredients:
- 5 oz   coix seed (Semen Coicis Lachryma-jobi, *yi yi ren*)
- 4 oz   beancurd stick (beancurd skin), cut into small pieces after soaking in water
- 10 pieces   ginko nuts, cut into halves
- 3 cups   water
-    rock sugar, desired amount to suit taste

After the soup boils, simmer for 2 to 3 hours. Add boiling water if more broth is desired. Consume all the ingredients.

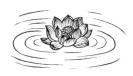

Chapter 9

Simple Solutions To
Health And Happiness

A long time ago, there was a wealthy merchant who lived in a big city. He could not understand why with the great wealth he possessed, his family had all deserted him. He was leading a lonely and unhappy life. When he needed company, he would invite his friends over. After the meat and wine were consumed, they all departed and he would seldom hear from them again. The merchant learned about a wise hermit living on top of a mountain. He went there to seek help. "What can I do to live a happier life?" The hermit invited the merchant to stay in his small hut. The merchant had a chance to taste the simple life which he had never known before. Although it was hard work to chop wood to make the fire and to gather the wild mushrooms and fruits for meals, the merchant slowly appreciated the message that the hermit wanted to convey. He returned to the city with a newfound view of life. He did not have to look further for a solution to his problem. The answer lay within himself. The merchant simply needed to show more love and care for the people around him.

In this technological age when many things are accomplished by just pressing a button, we tend to forget who we are and where we came from. We face many fundamental problems, the recurring one being how to live a healthier and happier life. The solutions can be as fundamental as the problems. We may not need a new technology for a solution. Often, the answer is simple and within reach, if only we appreciate its value.

The human race has been fighting diseases since the beginning of history. Our ancestors relied on herbs against infection before the dawn of medical science. The medical value of natural herbs have not changed, although our perception of them may have changed as influenced by the advancement of modern science. Medical technology has largely eclipsed the ancient wisdom that gave birth to the methods of herbal cure and prevention which we have inherited today. While we continue to explore the benefits that modern science brings, we should not neglect the valuable knowledge of herbs passed down from previous generations, for doing so would be discarding our past wisdoms and rejecting our roots.

As a practitioner of Chinese medicine for sixty years, I have treated and cured countless patients in Asia and America using Chinese herbs. My patients and I are among the millions of witnesses to the effectiveness of Chinese herbs, their gentleness on the body, and their preventive value. That the herbs are not more widely accepted is perhaps due to the cultural barrier between East and West. Another reason is the scant scientific evidence that explains how herbs work in the body. But even while we await further scientific proof, the empirical evidence through the ages regarding the healing and preventive effects of herbs is overwhelming, enough to show that they do work. This book, then, is a testament to this fact.

Bibliography

Beijing Medical College. *Dictionary of Traditional Chinese Medicine.* U.S. edition. San Francisco: China Books & Periodicals, 1985.

Beinfield, Harriet, and Efrem Korngold. *Between Heaven and Earth.* New York: Ballantine Books, 1991.

Bensky, Dan, and Andrew Gamble. *Chinese Herbal Medicine: Materia Medica.* Seattle: Eastland Press, 1986.

Bloomfield, Frena. *Chinese Beliefs.* London: Arrow Books, 1983.

Cheng, Xinnong. *Chinese Acupuncture and Moxibustion.* Beijing: Foreign Language Press, 1987.

Garvey, Jack. *The Five Phases of Food.* Newtonville, MA: Wellbeing Books, 1985.

Hyatt, Richard. *Chinese Herbal Medicine.* New York: Schocken Books, 1978.

Leslie, Charles. *Asian Medical Systems.* Berkeley: University of California Press, 1976.

Lu, Henry. *Chinese System of Food Cures.* New York: Sterling, 1986.

Matsumoto, Kikko, and Stephen Birch. *Five Elements and Ten Stems.* Brookline, MA: Paradigm Publications, 1983.

Porkert, Manfred. *Essentials of Chinese Diagnostics.* Zurich: Chinese Medicine Publications, Ltd., 1983.

Reid, Daniel. *Chinese Herbal Medicine.* Boston: Shambhala Publications, Inc., 1987.

Veith, Ilza. *The Yellow Emperor's Classic of Internal Medicine.* Berkeley: University of California Press, 1972.

Wallnofer, Henrich, and Anna Von Rottauscher. *Chinese Folk Medicine.* New York: Crown Books, 1972.

Wiseman, Nigel, and Andrew Ellis. *Fundamentals of Chinese Medicine*. Brookline, MA: Paradigm Publications, 1985.

Yeung, Him-che. *Handbook of Chinese Herbs and Formulas*. 2 vols. Los Angeles: Institute of Chinese Medicine, 1985.

Yin, Huihe, et al. *Fundamentals of Traditional Chinese Medicine*. Beijing: Foreign Languages Press, 1992.

Resources

For obtaining Dr. Fung's herbal formulas in tablets, additional books about Chinese Medicine, or a referral to a licensed practitioner using herbs, contact:

Health Concerns
8001 Capwell Drive
Oakland, CA 94621
(510) 639–0280

Herbal training for health practitioners and lay persons:

Get Well Foundation
7172 Regional Street, #116
Dublin, CA 94568–2324

(*Note:* most of these classes are held in the San Francisco Bay Area.)

Those interested in becoming informed about health freedom issues contact:

Citizens for Health
P.O. Box 1195
Tacoma, WA 98401
(206) 922–2456

Index

About The Authors

D r. Fung Fung practiced Chinese herbal medicine for almost sixty years. Dr. Fung is also a permanent consultant for Health Concerns, where he shares his valuable experience and helps select the herbs used in Health Concerns' products. He graduated from the College of Chinese Medicine in Canton, China, in 1934. He practiced medicine in the College Hospital for three years until the Japanese occupation. In Hong Kong, Dr. Fung continued his medical practice in the Tung Wah Group of Hospitals for the next two years. In 1939, he left for Vietnam to join the Cantonese Hospital in Cholon where he served as a resident physician for six years. In 1945, Dr. Fung started his private practice in Cholon, where he was known as Phung Phong (the Vietnamese translation of his Chinese name). He was married and had four children. His medical career in Cholon spanned thirty years until it was interrupted by the worsening war situation. Dr. Fung and his family returned to Hong Kong in 1969 where he continued his private practice for another ten years. In 1979, Dr. Fung and his family immigrated to the United States. Dr. Fung continued his private practice in San Francisco and Oakland until his retirement in 1993.

The co-author of this book is Dr. Fung's son. John Fung graduated from the University of California at Berkeley in 1971 with a B.A. in Economics, from the University of Chicago in 1978 with an M.A. in Social Sciences, and from Stanford University in 1989 with an M.S. in Engineering. John has worked as an economist and computer engineer for the last twenty years. In his spare time, he has done extensive research on Chinese medicine under the guidance of his father. Presently, John operates a consulting firm in Saratoga, California.

Books Available From Get Well Foundation

Chinese Herbs in the Western Clinic

by Andrew Gaeddert $15.95

Chinese Herbs in the Western Clinic recommends formulas by a variety of manufacturers that have been successfully used with thousands of American patients suffering from immune, digestive, gynecological, respiratory disorders, and other commonly seen complaints such as allergies, anxiety, arthritis, back pain, headaches, injury, insomnia and stress. Disorders are alphabetized by Western conditions and indexed by traditional Chinese medical terminology for easy reference while patients are in the office. This book is designed for practitioners.

Sixty Years in Search of Cures

by Dr. Fung Fung and John Fung $15.95

Sixty years in Search of Cures is the autobiography of one of the world's most experienced herbalists, Dr. Fung Fung, who routinely saw 100-150 patients per day working in a hospital clinic. This master practitioner with experience in Canton, Hong Kong, Vietnam, and San Francisco, reveals important dietary and lifestyle habits for the general public and herbal prescriptions for the professional herbalist.

Send check or money order payable to Get Well. Include $2.00 per book shipping and handling. California residents add $1.32 sales tax per book. Please be sure to write your name and address clearly, and to specify the titles and quantities of each book you want. Allow 4 weeks for delivery.

For trade, bookstore, and wholesale inquiries, contact North Atlantic Books, P.O. Box 12327, Berkeley, CA 94701.

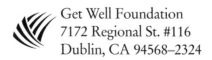

Get Well Foundation
7172 Regional St. #116
Dublin, CA 94568–2324